Chapter 1: Placebo Effect

About Placebos

Placebo is the typical term that is used to call a phony medication in the medical world. There are some placebos that are deliberately provided to the client to test or experiment some research. Nevertheless, there are also some variation of medications that are produced for the industrial requirements which include an incorrect or fake active ingredient. These types of medications can harm for your health and you really need to even more cautious in buying this item.

Comprehending the placebo will stop you from any possibilities of side-effects and any other more problems to your medication procedure. Rather than the components, this item also includes the incorrect dose that will be harming to you. If you want to stay away from placebo, you can attempt to buy the medication and any other drugs that you will consume in the pharmacy. This type of pharmacy will not sell any bad or poor-quality items of medications.

When you're buying them, you really need to double-check the medication that you purchase thoroughly. You can recognize the health factors of your medications by examining it well. You really need to check the register number of items that are generally released by the federal government. If you find the medication that is sold in inexpensive cost, you really need to reevaluate it right before acquiring it. If you find the exact same item, but it is offered at different rates, you really need to be even more cautious of these medication items as it can be a placebo. You will need to make certain the medication that you take is good, since it will straight affect your health.

Health Advantages

A recently released study of 679 internists and rheumatologists, chosen at random from a nationwide list, reports that over half of reacting doctors used incorrect medications - placebos - to deal with clients with difficult to treat conditions depending on the placebo effect to make them feel healthier. These doctors are making use of info that for a provided medical condition, it's not uncommon for one-third of clients to feel better after being treated with a placebo.

If you actually believe you will get much better, chances are, you will.
" Twenty to thirty percent of the advantages seen in rheumatism drug
research studies are because of the placebo effect. Genuine changes in health
support the belief that clients will get much better. Thanks to today's brain
images methods, the idea that ideas and beliefs impact your mental state, and
trigger the body to go through real natural changes has been revealed to be
real.

Understood to science as the placebo effect, this phenomenon has long been
observed in medical trials where clients who were taking a non-active
substance reported real enhancements, more enhancement than clients getting
no treatment at all. Placebos can either be a tablet made from non-active
compounds or a sham process meant to mimic the real one but without any
particular restorative activity that a client accepts as treatment. Any
subsequent healing influence is based upon the power of idea.

Using a placebo is a technique if a doctor is dealing with an issue that does
not have shown treatments. In spite of the drug businesses' best shots, brand-
new medications require time to develop, test and get to market. So many
conditions aren't totally comprehended or show different signs in different
people that you can see why dealing with a persistent issue can be a difficulty
for your physician.

According to the American Medical Association, using a placebo without
telling the client weakens trust and jeopardizes the relationship between
physician and client. The client ought to know if a drug is a placebo and
should never ever be given a prescription simply because they are viewed as
a tough or requiring client.

How do physicians clarify a placebo to clients? The AMA wants doctors to
tell clients that placebos aid better comprehend a condition by enabling them
to try different medications. Normally, a specialist will say something about
using a medication that's seldom used for your issue but may benefit you. If
you concur, the medical professional does not need to determine which
medication is a phony one.

If you're feeling a bit tricked by all of the, the physicians who follow this line of thinking fast to mention that they always have the best interest of the client at heart.

However, it's not unexpected that clients feel betrayed when they learn that they were handed a placebo, A delicate medical professional can clarify, "Simply because the placebo worked does not mean you're insane. You were in distress and therefore more vulnerable to responding to anything with the possible to help."

Do They Work?

Whenever a brand-new drug appears, scientists really need to perform tests so as to decide on its efficiency. In order to do so, they really need to compare the actual results with people who did not take the drug, but believe that they did. Bottom line, a group of people is split in 2 classifications: the ones in the very first series take the drug, while the other ones just believe that they have taken the drugs. The people taking part believe they take the real drug. The ones with placebos get a tablet that appears like the real drug, but includes no medication.

Research has revealed that there are certain situations in which a phony treatment, called a placebo, can be as reliable as real medication, as long as the people taking it do not know it's just a placebo. For instance, about 30-40% of clients struggling with conditions just like hypertension, arthritis, or perhaps Parkinson, show enhancement after taking placebo tablets. Furthermore, a fake surgical treatment, in which little cuts were made on client's knees, revealed the exact same actual results as real arthroscopic surgical treatment in one research study of arthritis treatment.

There's no outright truth concerning placebos. Nobody truly understands what happens when a placebo has a favorable medical impact. Nevertheless, it appears that placebos promote some sort of integrated recovery power of the brain. Your brain can release substances that have comparable results to those of morphine, and research studies have revealed that, under certain conditions, these substances are released by the brain if the client actually believes that a tablet will eliminate strong pain. That way, the brain substances have the exact same impact as pain reliever.

When scientists need to identify the efficiency of a brand-new drug, they compare the real influence of the proposed drug with the placebo effect. If the drug is not more reliable than the placebo, it means that it has no real impact.

There's a great series of effects in which placebos can do the thing they need to, enabling your brain to take control of the real pain. Nevertheless, placebos do not always work. Unlike those conditions where the brain appears to have untapped resources, more serious illnesses like cancer do not react to placebos.

Is It a Triumph of the Mind?

A placebo effect is recovery based entirely on the power of recommendation, not on the action of an active chemical compound. A placebo, in some cases called a "sugar tablet", is made to appear like a "real drug" and provokes restorative impacts when administered, regardless of its absence of any kind of active compound.

But, please, do not deceive yourself. It's insufficient to take a "sugar tablet" and expect a placebo effect. No, you also really need the recommendation, from an authority figure, that the tablet will assist in recovery. Somebody who can make you really believes in it. The crucial point is not the tablet; it is the tips and expectations. You really need to rely on the authority first, and after that to accept that "the tablet" will actually help you. Belief, inspiration, and expectation are necessary to the placebo effect.

What is the belief? The belief is that you have the capability to make something happen. This belief in one's proficiency for healing is a really strong predictor for recuperating from any illness. There is a well-known saying that the effectiveness of the treatment depends, not so much on the doctor's proficiency, but rather on the doctor's selflessness and empathy. The placebo effect contributes in the empathy, not in the competence.

What does placebo represent, anyhow? Remarkably, it represents the Latin expression: "I will please" One clarification says that every little thing began when somebody came for a treatment which did not exist, yet the medical professional wanted to please the client. So he offered the client something that he actually knew was inefficient, but said that it worked in treatment.

Clearly, this medical professional was somebody well knowledgeable about the mind/ body connection and the results of the positive thinking. The medical professional knew: I really need to persuade my client of the treatment's efficiency. I really need to have fun with the client's mindset and his/her capability to recover. He knew that the client would only "feel better" but would not be much healthier.

The accomplishment of mind and belief over body? Yes, and researchers are well aware of the power of mind over body. If clients really believe in a treatment, they can enhance their medical condition. What science says is: beliefs, suggestibility and hopes about treatment might use biochemistry of our bodies. We know that ideas can impact brain neurochemistry, and that the human neurochemical system is impacted by other biochemical systems (hormonal/immune). We are our ideas. What we really need to learn much from all these descriptions is: sensory experience and ideas can impact neurochemistry. Positive thinking can generate real neurochemical reactions in the body.

The next time you have a health problem; remember that your confident mindset and beliefs might be extremely essential to your healing from injury or disease. Optimism, positive thinking, an enthusiastic mindset and genuine belief, are all really fundamental parts of your body's battle against disease. There is no secret: positive thinking works. Now we know. The capability of the mind to produce recovery changes depends upon emotions, and can affect physical health for better or even worse.

Can you really believe that half of a drug's impacts are because of the placebo reaction? Sapirstein, who evaluated 39 research studies, done between 1974 and 1995, of depressed clients treated with drugs, psychiatric therapy, or a mix of both. He found that half of the drug impact was because of the placebo reaction. Yet, there are a lot of research studies that have found unbiased enhancements in health from placebos to support the idea that the placebo effect is completely mental. The placebo effect is a recovery procedure, not just a treating one. Recovery changes both mind and body on a deep level. We are driven by our minds, by idea, by expectations.

Regrettably, we are likewise driven by worry and incorrect expectations. As an ill person, a client pleads for understanding and empathy, "asking" for a comparable reaction from medical workers. For that reason, instructors teach our healthcare specialists to show attention, care, love, and hope when they are dealing with an ill man or woman. As clients, we really need to rely on our own capability for healing, in any given treatment, medication or process and, most importantly, in our health therapists. Even just remaining in the recovery circumstance achieves something.

If you have any ethical issues, just like "with placebos, we are selling incorrect hope and magic treatments for all health problem" you do not really need to stress. There are different unobservable procedures that presumably perform all sorts of magic analgesic and alleviative functions, in the exact same way as "sugar tablets". A lot of doubters will turn down faith, hope, belief and even alternative medical practices just like homeopathy. We know that they might not treat cancer, but by promising and alleviating distress, placebos can supply some step of convenience. Giving some convenience in a completely awkward circumstance is another reason to support the declaration:" What distinction does it make why something works, as long as it appears to work? ".

As always, we, as human society, really need to be crucial in our method to the placebo. We do not want to see the placebo as an open door to quackery, nor for huge dishonest company. Our intent is to safeguard innocent people from charlatans, exposing the door to alternative treatments.

The Law of Attraction

If you give sugar tablets to a group of clients and tell them that these tablets are going to treat them, some of them will actually get much better. This is understood in the medical world as the placebo effect. Every physician, nurse and medical student know about it, but no-one has had the ability to clarify it.

To put it just, the placebo effect suggests that if you really believe a specific treatment will work for you, it generally does.

Let me show you an example.
Several years ago, a young heart cosmetic surgeon from Seattle by the name of Leonard Cobb performed an uncommon experiment. He carried out certain fake surgical treatments on clients struggling with angina. Rather than carrying out real surgical treatments, he just made the cut and after that sewed

it back together. He didn't actually do anything that could provide any sort of treatment, but remarkably, 90% of the clients reported that the process helped. The sham operations showed to be just as efficient as the real ones.

Isn't that incredible? The clients were not treated by the surgical treatments - they were treated by their belief in the surgical treatment. Here are more instances:

In one research study, medical professionals removed warts by utilizing the power of belief. They painted them with common red color and told the clients that when the color wears away, the warts will vanish.

In a research study of asthmatics, scientists found that they could produce dilation of the respiratory tracts by telling people they were breathing in bronchodilators, even when they weren't.
With using the brain images strategies, physicians had the ability to show that ideas and beliefs can actually trigger the body to go through real natural changes.

The simple fact is, that if we really actually believe in something, we have the capability to treat (or perhaps hurt) ourselves. This is a well-known simple fact in today's medication. Herbert Benson from Harvard University revealed that the placebo effect operates in as much as 60-90% of illnesses, consisting of angina pectoris, bronchial asthma, herpes simplex, and duodenal ulcers.

On the other hand, the presently well-known law of attraction declares that if you really actually believe into something, you can 'draw in' it into your life. Make it your reality through the power of belief. So if you really believe that a specific treatment will make you better, the law of attraction claims that it will.

Obviously, when it pertains to our own bodies, the law of attraction is absolutely nothing more than some variation of the placebo effect. In simple fact, some people would reach to declare that the placebo effect itself is a certain evidence for the efficiency of the law of attraction. While this is true, in my viewpoint, taking it a bit too far, it is intriguing to keep in mind that the law of attraction can in fact, at the very least partly, work.

How to Use These Concepts
Both the placebo effect and the law of attraction could and most likely should

be used in medication. Numerous scientific research studies have revealed the efficiency of the placebo effect and just dismissing it since it's not a 'real' medication would be really wrong. There is, nevertheless, one issue.

If a client understands that all he's getting is a sweet tablet, there is no simple way for him to persuade himself that this treatment will really work. As a result, the treatment will undoubtedly struggle to work. If, on the other hand, we choose to lie to the client and tell him that what he's getting is the real remedy, we are dealing with a major ethical problem.

Just because of that issue, the placebo effect and the law of attraction are presently not being applied in any traditional medication. What could potentially be the most flexible of all remedies - the supreme 'magic tablet' - is being neglected since none of us has managed to determine how to use it. We can only hope that the present interest surrounding the law of attraction will bring us some brand-new insight and potentially show us a much different method to utilizing this effective concept.

Is It the Supplement or Your Mind Working?

Back throughout The Second World War, the medics and healthcare facilities would usually run out of pain relievers and would give their clients the most recent and biggest pain reliever, comfort.

In some cases, they would inject the soldiers with what they were told to be morphine, but was actually a healthy dosage of saline resolution, or saltwater. The bright side is that, when injected with the "morphine," the majority of the soldiers' strong pain would disappear, at least for a little while.

The Placebo Effect
The medics weren't precisely fooling the soldiers; they were triggering a placebo effect. The placebo effect is essentially a series of responses in the brain that can change its mental or physiological performance. Like in the example of the soldiers, they thought they were getting morphine, which they know dulls the strong pain instantly, but they were given saltwater. The response was the exact same; it counteracted the strong pain, at least temporarily. The reason for this is since your brain manages your body, and your mind can unconsciously manage your brain.

Bodybuilding Placebo Impacts

The placebo effect overflows into the muscle getting environment through other drugs referred to as supplements. The truth is tons of the supplements on the racks do not actually include any active components that would trigger somebody to get muscle. Some supplements are a lot like a shot of saltwater; they are worthless and just get performed. Other supplements have really little active component, but inadequate to represent any muscle development that somebody may experience while on the supplement.

Many muscle getting hopefuls do not just walk into a shop and buy any fancy tub of powder they see. They generally make "notified" choices based upon what they have read in publications or spoken with other ones. Most of the times, when somebody begins taking a dietary supplement for the first time, it's a leap of faith. They are using the supplement for one basic reason, since they really believe it will work.

The belief is crucial here. When you really believe something totally, and back it with feeling, you can achieve things that once appeared unrealistic. This consists of physiological changes, or changes to the body. By thinking and thinking that the supplement that was just taken in will trigger muscle development, the brain takes it as directions. Generally, just because of the person's strong conviction, the person's brain will actually get to work and begin the bodybuilding procedure. It will do this since it was told to do it.

Now, generally when a student begins a brand-new supplement, they actually believe it will help build muscle. With every little thing else staying the exact same, this belief is strong enough to stimulate development. The thing is how many people begin a brand-new supplement and keep doing what they are doing? Very few. Many people will get on the "brand-new wonder" and will kick their training up a notch. Not only will they enhance their training, they typically enhance their nutrition and healing.

Give Yourself Some Credit

If you were to make those enhancements to your muscle getting technique: training more strongly, eating better, and resting appropriately, would not you acquire muscle anyhow, even without the supplement? The answer is a definite yes. A lot of people get on a supplement and give all credit for enhancement to the supplement. Provide yourself more credit. You did the work, not the supplement. Chances are, the supplement didn't even do anything, and it was just a placebo. Some supplements are well worth taking and do the body some great, but if you do not build the structure with strong training, nutrition, healing ... the supplements will not do you any great. Now if supplements can't help build muscle with poor training and nutrition, do you believe they aid with appropriate training and nutrition? Perhaps a little, but it's you are getting the actual results, not the supplement.

Here are 3 simple steps to wean yourself off of unneeded supplements:

1. Gradually stop using whatever you want to quit and see your actual results not slip, but actually believe that they will enhance. Apply the placebo effect for your benefit.

2. Understand that it's you are doing the effort, not the supplement. So give yourself the credit.

3. Start thinking in yourself and your capability to get muscle. Just as a belief in a supplement can trigger development, actually believe in yourself and see what happens.

Now you can use the placebo effect to your benefit and use your mind and muscle connection to build muscle.

The Relationship to Objectives

The placebo effect is a very real thing. Many research studies validate that when a client is given a placebo or "sugar tablet rather than medication and told it was the remedy to their specific condition, they were usually spontaneously recovered. That is the power of the mind to recover the body. When an individual actually believes the placebo to be a real remedy and expects it to be so, the body reacts appropriately. The body is simply taking orders from the brain.

So what does this have to do with your objectives? A lot actually. When you set an objective, and I mean a BIG objective, do you really believe it will pertain to fulfillment? Are you definitely sure it will happen without a shadow of a doubt? Do you expect it to be effective? Like the man or woman taking the placebo, you need to really believe in your objectives and realize that you will accomplish them with unwavering expectations.

Sadly, as the majority of us know, when we make the exact same New Year's resolutions each year, we are still wishing for the wanted result, but are certainly not sure anymore that it's possible. We are most likely to really believe a physician who we barely know that he has the cure-all to make us better, than we are to actually believe in ourselves and our capability to produce the life we prefer.

Sure, a medical professional is the specialist in the field of health, but you are the professional of your own life. If you really need a specialist to tell you your dreams are now coming to life, then look to the greatest authority of all-deep space, God, Infinite intelligence, whatever you choose to call this higher power. Having faith that you are being supported and expecting the actual results you want is a lot like taking a placebo.

The opposite of the placebo effect is the nocebo influence. A nocebo influence is an ill influence triggered by the idea or belief that something is hazardous. To put it simply, the only limitations we need to attain our objectives are the ones our company believe in. Tons of those beliefs have been hardwired into subconscious. If we find ourselves hesitating or self-sabotaging our objectives, then we have an unconscious belief that the objective is not possible-contradicting our desire. These kinds of beliefs usually are available in the form of "recommendations" offered to us by other ones (mother and father, authority figures, instructors) that we adopt and really believe as our truth, like "You will never ever amount to anything" or "Who do you believe you are to really want that?"

People say "I'll actually believe it when I see it", but the truth is, they will see it when they actually believe it purposely and automatically. An objective is attained when it is totally heeded with the power of faith and expectations. This is where wonders happen. Faith is a location in your heart where you rely on yourself and the future, not the ideas of other ones -it's where great objective accomplishments are possible.

Placebo in Medical Care

The positive influence of placebo is clear in tons of regions of life, not the least of which is in healthcare. Precisely how this operates in the procedure of recovery relationships and encounters with healthcare service providers remains mostly undeveloped and inadequately comprehended. Ideally clients enhance after checking out a healthcare supplier as a result of particular treatment. If treatment is medication or surgical treatment, it is simpler to comprehend and gauge the procedure and scientific result.

The nature of tons of conditions, even cancer or serious mental illness, is to enhance spontaneously and rather unexpectedly. The best example of placebo effect is the double-blind drug research study. We know the control group in drug research studies is given a "blank" tablet where neither the person giving the tablet nor the recipient understands whether it is a placebo or the active medication. General 25-30% of research study individuals will see beneficial actual results with placebo.

This translates as many individuals in medical practice will get a lot better if given the very wrong drug, for the very wrong reason, at the very wrong time. The doctor might too advise the client to do something worthless like stand in the corner for 3 minutes two times daily and have as much success with their signs enhancing. The main point is that the impact of placebo is a crucial yet improperly comprehended and very likely underutilized phenomenon.

It has actually been said that there is most likely a physiologic clarification for this instead of it being a random event. Undoubtedly with our minimal grasp of brain function, placebo effect or the belief that something great is going to happen very likely take advantage of certain biochemical paths in the brain that improve the gut feeling of well being and even have a direct impact on the body immune system. What needs more attention is what element of the recovery encounter promotes these paths? This is actually true for sees with the medical care doctor, other healthcare companies, psychological health professional, therapist, good friend, or really loved ones.

The person needs a much better grasp of their condition. Info that clarifies plainly what is going on should start to improve convenience and relief. Understanding what they are up against and getting rid of the unidentified helps immeasurably. If the person feels that there is a collaboration with their medical care company who reveals caring issue for their predicament, it supports a favorable mindset in the client. The above info makes it possible for a sense of control or proficiency over the condition. It at the minimum supplies a structure of stability from which the client can start to compete with the condition. Talk treatment and teaching the standard concepts of mindfulness can help concentrate on the job at hand.

Promoting clear thinking re: what is necessary and engaging, while neglecting the illogical or mind-blowing, can make the distinction in how the client feels about their present condition and in being an active certified individual in the healing procedure. The more notified, supported and empowered the client is made to feel, the more reliable the treatment will be. How to link the dots to make all of our relationships more recovery needs more research study and practice. It will certainly expose a wealth of untapped resources.

Placebo and Weight-loss

Weight reduction is an uphill struggle for many. In a world where there is an increasing need for instantaneous services, weight-loss items appear to take advantage of it. With anything from weight reduction spots to wonder berries and even cosmetic surgery. All of us want to look great and with publication covers plastered with ultra slim models we are all sensation that really need to look great. Sadly reality doesn't enable us to put in the time and effort to eat well, to get the workout and to normally give the time and attention to reduce weight and keep it off.

Among the most neglected parts of weight-loss relates to this exceptionally effective idea of The Placebo effect. In simple fact, lots of trick weight-loss items actually has The Placebo effect to believe for its success. It's a remarkable event and its bee n shown over and over again in double blind research studies in essentially every medical field.

It highlights the significance of our beliefs and how your belief are effective adequate to effect any change in your body. In essence, The Placebo Impact is the influence that your mind needs to persuade your body to attain a wanted impact. In its preliminary research studies, it was shown that sugar tablets that have no medical homes have precisely the exact same impact as strong drugs - as long as the client beliefs that the tablet will have a specific influence.

Not only has this turned the medical community on its head, it's actually opened us op to an entire brand-new field to check out. The mind truly is more effective than what we tend to really believe. It ends up that medication is not actually essential at all, but what's truly needed is the belief. When it concerns weight-loss, its amazing how many obese people really believe that they can't drop weight; that it's in their "genes" and that they have tried "every little thing". The simple fact of the matter is that when you change your mind and when you change your beliefs, anything is possible.

Wrinkle Creams

In the research study of anti aging, there are plainly specified lines between the most effective wrinkle creams and one that show no actual results. And while we expect to see radiant evaluations from the best wrinkle creams, we do not expect the exact same from ones that revealed no lead to scientific research studies, yet radiant evaluations still exist. For many years, this irregular event was believed to be because of marketing efforts till a research study analyzed the placebo effect of wrinkle creams.

For those of you who do not comprehend what is meant by placebo effect of wrinkle creams, its describing the simple fact that lots of people show arise from wrinkle creams just since they really believe it works, not as the cream itself works. The placebo effect is not separated only to wrinkle creams in simple fact the broad spread usage of "sugar tablets" or sham surgical treatments are other typical examples of the power of the placebo effect. People can just start to show indications of recovery since they actually believe that whatever they are taking is assisting them. A sugar tablet might be alternatived to medication since the client doesn't actually really need medication, but they believe that they do. By supplying clients a "solution" they can take, they start to feel better and really believe that they are being treated of whatever was ailing them.

When it concerns wrinkle creams, there is no objective to offer customers an incorrect or fake wrinkle treatment nevertheless there are a lot of inefficient wrinkle creams out there. Customers though might feel so highly about the efficiency of the creams and serums that they actually start to show indications of recovery wrinkles. Due to the fact that the brain plays such a crucial role in the recovery of the physique, if it really believes that it is getting what it needs, it assists in the recovery of the skin. This impact has been shown in tons of elements of the medical field, but is only now being realized by anti aging specialists. Despite how efficient a wrinkle cream might be great lines and wrinkles can be smoothed and filled just as customers really believe that they are getting an efficient treatment.

The weird feature of wrinkle creams that is different than lots of examples of the placebo effect in medication is that there is a comparable event that happens even when the wrinkle creams being used program incredible lead to scientific research studies. The customers who actually believe in the wrinkle creams efficiency show better actual results than the customers who are hesitant. While this would not be certified as an example of the placebo effect per say, it is the power of positive thinking that engages the brain to help in the treatment of wrinkle cream. This is a fascinating idea in the anti aging market since people have such differing viewpoints about which wrinkle creams work the best, when it appears that as long as you are using an efficient cream that you entire heartedly actually believe is working, you skin will show indications of enhancement.

The power of the brain is plainly incredible, and the placebo effect is definitely an example of that. Whether applied to recovering the physique in medication and even something as easy as a wrinkle cream, the capability of your brain to recover your body is interesting to say the least. Individuals have gotten rid of serious illnesses by staying positive, or not "letting the illness beat them." We usually come up with this as positive thinking and luck that is directing these strong willed people to their survival, though when taken into the setting of the placebo effect, you need to really wonder what role that is playing in the recovery of these people.

When it concerns recovery wrinkles, it is not a matter of life and death and yet the brain still has the capability to recover such signs. When you actually believe that you have found the best wrinkle cream and you use it with positivity, your wrinkles truly do disappear. If you follow that reasoning and you research and are certain that you have found the absolute best that the anti aging market needs to provide, your actual results would be significantly enhanced by thinking entire heartedly that you have found the resolution for your wrinkles. Wrinkle creams can do remarkable things by themselves nowadays, but they can barely touch the confusion efficient in the brain with just a little belief.

Reducing High Blood Pressure

The Placebo effect is when a phony medication, treatment or process is provided to an unknowing client and it produces the exact same actual results as a genuine treatment. This been of interest to science for several years. For people wishing to enhance their health, minimize high blood pressure, and change their way of life, the placebo effect has tons of useful ramifications.

What can we learn much from it? The real lesson can be summarized in Robert Wiseman's 59 seconds "By advising the attendants of the amount of workout they handled a day-to-day basis, they changed their beliefs about themselves, and their bodies reacted to make these brand-new beliefs a truth ... so simply thinking of your typical everyday workout can make you healthier."

This experiment shows the power of human beliefs, giving the worn out old PMA expression 'what you actually believe you can accomplish' a brand-new lease of life. If somebody can slim down and lower their high blood pressure just since they change their belief to believe they are residing in a much healthier way, when in actuality absolutely nothing had changed, we can then comprehend that we do manifest our ideas in our physiques.

If the reverse had happened, and the attendants were told they were leading unhealthy lives it follows that the attendants would have gained weight and suffered poorer health, just because of proof of what they were concentrating on. This is essential. The cleaners were not only outlined their healthy way of lives once, but asked to gauge and evaluate their calorie burn, and do so frequently. This conduct strengthened the brand-new belief that their jobs were healthy and great quantifiable actual results followed.

The most crucial thing we can draw from this is that the beliefs we handle are as crucial as the physical scenarios we are in. For that reason, when you are thinking negative ideas, you are might unknowingly become the author of negative effect in your life. Changing our beliefs includes some discipline, but as tons of us know, once practices are formed, they are tough to break. So let us form some great ones now:

In addition to your healthy way of life:

take a journal and note how many times you are physically active when you walk, or do the household chores, or climb up the stairs. If you will not do this, at least log it in your mind and praise yourself on such healthy efforts. This will pay the exact same weight decreasing, high blood pressure reducing dividends similar to the hotel attendants.

Beyond your circulatory health, if you can choose to really believe better about yourself, that you are a really good person efficient in considerable accomplishment, then you can produce it. If you can really believe you are positive, then you can produce those actual results.
You have within you the secrets to of ending up being every little thing you want to be. It begins with declining to handle the negative, and instead choosing what you really want that is great. You are more control than you believe.

Does It Associate with Hypnosis?

A crucial thing to keep in mind is that you can get in a hypnotic trance just as much when you're negative as when you're positive. If you have permitted yourself to believe only the absolute worst about any circumstance, the majority of particularly yourself; you can never ever pass examinations, you're worthless at this, you can't do that, and so on, then your impulses are configured in an unfavorable way.

The common argument used by pessimists is the one about; "Well, I'm only being a realist. Things actually are that bad." Do not forget that expectation is an effective tool. By continuously thinking the worst, you have configured your brain into expecting the worst.

This concept is really effective. Your mindsets in life are determined by how effective your unconscious expectations are. Any medical professional will tell you, if he's being sincere, that expectations can even treat disease. For this reason, placebos.

You might remember that we showed using placebos once in a short article on a chap who was suffering stress and anxiety attacks. They make very first rate anti-depressants. If you have a favorable belief that a sugar tablet will work, though at the time you're uninformed that it's a sugar tablet, the span produced by the positive belief in the tablet's effectiveness will produce positive actual results.

Where hypnosis is so practical is that it's a medium, a channel if you like, through which you can program and preserve positive subconscious span. The more your attention is engaged and your attention locked onto the placebo, the more effective it will be. It'll actually re-organize the cellular structure in your body.

The completion of the span is the success of the placebo, and this naturally is the hypnotic angle. The way a placebo tablet works is because of the post-hypnotic reaction, which regrettably few physicians comprehend, or are prepared to admit.

If you actually believe naturally that things are going to work out well, then your self-confidence will stay high and for that reason you'll have a lot more staying power to see the job through. Your energy and interest, too, will be a lot higher, which in turn will stimulate other ones, if you're operating in a group.

You'll find that you'll begin to produce services obviously out of nowhere at all with a stream of ideas, since your subconscious will be continuously working toward manifesting your expectations. Keep in mind how effective your brain is, and it's definitely important that it's directed to what will be useful for you.

A good deal of research has been done in this field, and it's been revealed that optimists live longer, suffer less tension and have better body immune systems. Just because of their inherent self-confidence, then, they'll stand firm and are even more very likely to be successful.

When a Placebo Isn't Real

Usually when standard innovations flop to work it's not unusual for a brand-new treatment to be dismissed as "it's the placebo effect", if it helps the client. This is so extremely typical with the persistent real pain client and could potentially be the even worse usage of the term "placebo" in medication and regulative parlance.

Here's some background on the course the persistent real pain client takes. The strong pain could be of "unidentified etiology" or it could be an illness procedure like fibromyalgia, RSD, Carpal Tunnel Syndrome, or the typical secondary medical diagnosis of sciatica. The problem however is clear. The sign has ended up being the medical diagnosis just since the client's issue cannot be fixed and the strong pain is not gotten rid of.

Prior to the medical diagnosis progressing to "persistent real pain" the client displays her/himself as a client that has come for medical attention because of strong pain. The preliminary test usually includes an initial medical diagnosis being made and after that a treatment procedure is developed for that client. Most of the times like extending disc, degenerative disc illness, Tic Doloreux as examples there is a physical reason for the strong pain and if that is found through laboratory tests, radiology, observation and so on then the reason for the strong pain is found and dealt with. The real pain disappears since the causative aspect is found and dealt with, or the cause is determined and the client is informed that it could be a viral causation and, time, is the therapist with treatment only for the symptomatic real pain till the infection is gone or the condition is untreatable.

In the majority of circumstances, it will be something easy to eliminate the issue just like prescription antibiotics, anti-inflammatory, aspirin, ibuprofen, rest, hot/cold techniques, or physical treatment. The real pain sign disappears, and the medical group no longer sees the client since there is no issue. Cause has been dealt with and real pain is no longer present. Client is "well".

Nevertheless, there are a particular portion of the above clients that the treatment procedure did not work. Those clients did every little thing they were told to do yet the strong pain continues, and they continue to check out the medical professional grumbling the real pain is not improving and might actually be worsening. If the physician is a medical care doctor it is now the client is referred out to some other specialized just like neurology, rheumatology, orthopedics, neurosurgery, chiropractic or another person. New evaluates start, evaluation of old tests continues and the dealing with medical professional understands, or should know, the conventional solutions did not work. A crucial indicate keep in mind is when the client has reached this point in the treatment of "real pain" the success rate at this moment for these clients is 0 %. It is no longer legitimate to state that "80% of these clients get even better with bed rest and aspirin". These clients did not.

If the client continues to experience strong pain any prior medical diagnosis might be eliminated, and a brand-new medical diagnosis arises. The brand-new "medical diagnosis" is "persistent strong pain" perhaps "due to", or "of unidentified etiology". It is this time that the medical occupation and other alternative specialists admit the reason the client is experiencing strong pain is "unidentified or untreatable".

This is where making use of the term "placebo" is lost or misused. At this moment in time the prior declarations about how clients that have been dealt with effectively blur the reality that the persistent client has been down the standard course, unsuccessfully, so now the client population is significantly different than the clients who were dealt with effectively. It is no longer legitimate to referral treatments following this phase to be revealed as being "placebo". It is better for our comprehending to advance the principle those treatments now that work might be because of our misconceptions, instead of the fall back expression "placebo". Anything that stops the real pain is a treatment method that is brand-new and has a favorable result when all former treatments stopped working.

It's so typical for positive treatment results to be crossed out as "placebo", even if only a sugar tablet, but the objective of all people who choose to help other individuals is to accomplish the objectives of assisting by stopping the condition. With persistent strong pain clients the condition is "continuing, persistent strong pain".

Are there quacks? Yes. Are there shysters? Yes. Are there those who declare to deal with, accept cash for doing so, yet do not. Yes.

It's better to try to comprehend and to not accept prejudicial declarations when by trying to comprehend and clarify properly would better serve the persistent real pain client.

Better Than Drugs

Over the past thirty years or so, efficiency boosting drugs have ended up being the standard for lots of professional athletes. Professional athletes are more powerful, much faster, they can last longer, and a lot of them associate drugs to these advances in efficiency. According to certain researchers nevertheless, drugs have little to do with the increased efficiency. Instead it is all in the professional athlete's mind.

A current double-blind trial financed by the World Anti-Doping Company tested 2 groups of people. The very first group were given a dosage of human development hormonal agent and the 2nd group were given a placebo. Neither the individuals nor the scientists knew who got which.

The scientists then asked individuals to think whether they were on the real drug. Incredibly, the group that got the placebo but that thought they had gotten the drug enhanced in their efficiency on 4 considerable steps - sprint capability, endurance, power, and strength.

This was in contrast to the individuals who got the placebo but had thought properly that they got the placebo. Ken Ho, an endocrinologist who led the research study said that "This finding actually shows the power of the mind".

Ken is precisely right. Tons of professional athletes are taking drugs, but a ton of the results of the drugs aren't the drugs themselves but rather what the professional athlete is thinking the drugs should do to their efficiency.

Another component that enhances this simple fact is that in a different double-blind research study, human development hormonal agent was not considered to be handy at all with increasing efficiency. The professional athletes who got the drug did not get any benefit since they did not actually believe the drug would provide any benefit.

The placebo effect is typically understood amongst researchers but not amongst the public and professional athletes. Time and time again research studies have revealed that it is the power of the mind and belief that can materialize changes in individuals' capability, and it has extremely little to do with drugs and supplements.

Professional athletes these days and of the future need to take this info seriously and to train their minds as much as they train their bodies. As the controller of our own minds, we actually have the power to direct our body can doing.

Self-belief is just something that all the best professional athletes worldwide share. Science is beginning to show us that perhaps it is this self-belief that has lead these professional athletes to the top, and not just because of they are born with some inherent skill to be the best.

Root-Cause Hypnotherapy and the Placebo effect

A typical method in scientifically-based "double-blind" tests to establish the credibility of a treatment or a drug includes using a placebo. This is basically a neutral compound which does not achieve anything in and of itself. Analogically, an individual's simple "belief" in the effectiveness of a provided treatment or a drug can be said to be as a result of a "placebo effect."

With this in mind, it is very important to deal with the reasonable issue relating to Origin Hypnotherapy and whether placebo effect can contribute in it - or undoubtedly in hypnotherapy in general.

Placebo effect remains among the largest puzzles in modern-day medication and psychology alike.

Why? As, undoubtedly and to the distress of nearly everybody - it works regularly than it does not. Double-blind tests regularly use placebos to evaluate the effectiveness of brand-new drugs. In lots of such tests, placebos perform precisely as can be expected, i.e. they accomplish precisely absolutely nothing, and hence the given drug can be efficiently tested for its effectiveness and capability to deal with the given condition.

But there is also a "dark side" here - or at least a really strange side. There are many cases where a placebo works - or does not - in specific reverse of what reasoning would determine.

Cases where a client is given a specific drug and told that it's a placebo - can extremely usually lead to an unanticipated outcome: the client, who knows what the drug "must" do, yet now "understands" that he/she is taking a placebo ... does not respond to the drug.

Opposite cases where the client is given a placebo, but is told that it's the real thing, then understanding what the "expected" result ought to be - the client complies. Not intentionally, mind you. His/her BODY complies.

Explores alcohol have been performed where groups of people were given non-alcoholic drinks and were asked to get intoxicated. They did. Some of them got absolutely delirious too.

With all this in mind, it would be disingenuous of me to unconditionally dismiss the possibility of a placebo effect at work in hypnotherapy in general or Source Hypnotherapy in specific.

Anxiety Treatments

A Placebo is a pharmaceutical preparation which contains no active components. Those who are given a placebo might feel relief just as they believe they are actually getting medication. It improves their general impact and addresses the desire for medication. On the other hand, administering a placebo to a client is also used to meet the therapists' requirement to treat their clients. Placebos are also normal used in research studies evaluating the efficiency of medications.

In dealing with anxiety, research studies have been done to see what the real impacts of placebo treatments for anxiety are by doing brain imaging research studies. Brain imaging tests real changes in the blow flow in the brain of those taking placebos that was noticeably comparable to what those taking antidepressants experienced. Other research studies really believe that over 70% of the effective usage of antidepressant medication is due more to the "placebo effect" than the anti-depressant treatment.

Just like some common medications when they are stopped, the client actually experiences physical signs of withdrawal as the drugs leave their body. Those who got placebo treatments for anxiety also experienced such withdrawal signs. Hormonal agent Replacement Treatment research studies revealed that when taken off of the medication, nearly half of the grievances was associated with strong pain and tightness. Musculoskeletal problems were the 2nd most typical grievance of those getting placebo treatments followed by fatigue.

In order for placebo treatments for anxiety, or any other health issue to work, the person getting the placebo (also called a "sugar tablet") should not know they are getting it. This is called the 'Span Influence' it a mindful and unconscious control of the client using classical conditioning. This is the procedure where a stimulus produces a particular reaction. The client then associates a stimulus (placebo treatment) to feeling relief similar way as clients taking real medication expect relief.

No matter the kind of treatment for anxiety that is used, in most cases they work. Not every medication or placebo will work for everybody. It is always best to seek advice from your doctor about any medication you may be thinking about. Treatments are readily available and lots of turn to natural treatments that are particularly created to resolve the particular signs of depressive conditions. The solution is normally created in oral dietary supplements.

The greatest quality supplements are of pharmaceutical grade and the metabolic course of the active ingredients will have been tested at the molecular level. Also, the interaction of the active ingredients is tested. This procedure lets you know you are getting the active ingredients the label says you are and that you are getting the best quality supplement.

Recovering Metals and Rocks

It has been said for centuries that by wearing copper, an individual can minimize or remove strong pain connected with swelling and arthritis. Baseball gamers have begun sporting lockets made from titanium as it is thought that this metal will support the body's energy flow. Gold and silver, which are 2 well-known metals in the precious jewelry creation market, are supposed to have powers that can recover the body and assistance make the most of cognitive functions in the brain. Can wearing a copper bracelet actually lower the strong pain of arthritis or do the bracelets just wind up being another quite piece of precious jewelry?

A research study suggests that those who wear copper and magnetic bracelets aren't getting any fringe benefits from doing so. The research study also suggests that if people who wear copper and magnetic bracelets for their recovery powers might feel less strong pain, but only because of mental results. What this means is that the positive side results being felt by those who wear these bracelets are basically experiencing a placebo effect.

For those not acquainted with the placebo effect, the medical field uses it to try and figure out whether a medication or gadget is really assisting people. For instance, when evaluating brand-new medications, pharmaceutical businesses will typically give some clients real medication and only give other clients a placebo. This placebo is normally a sugar tablet which consists of no medication in it at all. It is also kept a secret to the individuals of the research study concerning what tablet they were actually given. At the end of the research study, those given the placebo tablet often report that their condition had enhanced, but in all truth, their enhancement was mental and not physical.

Still, some argue that it needs to not matter whether it can be shown whether wearing metals actually enhances an individual's condition. Those who actually believe in metal treatment say that if it helps the client or person than that's all that should matter. Doubters point out nevertheless that there are certain people that should not be exposed to magnets. Individuals with pacemakers, who are pregnant, wear medication spots or use an insulin pump should keep away from magnets as they might hinder the condition an individual has or the medical gadgets that they use.

Right before modern-day medication happened, silver was usually use as an antimicrobial representative and as a disinfectant. In health shops and on the Web, colloidal silver is being sold and many individuals are purchasing it up. Colloidal silver is when small particles are suspended in liquid and the FDA alerts that customers should stay far. Those who use colloidal silver over an extended period of time can trigger argyria, and this makes an individual's skin turn a grayish-blue color. For those with this condition, it cannot be reversed, and they are actually stuck to a very different skin color for the rest of their lives. Silver can also trigger stomach issues and kidney damage.

While there are no tested claims of metals or magnets that will treat conditions or deal with disorders, customers still acquire metal products, supplements and fashion jewelry including magnetic parts in hopes that it will work for them. Present medications and treatments for arthritis are usually costly and do little to reduce the strong pain that is related to the illness.

Chapter 2: Subconscious Thinking

Every little thing that happens in our life is affected by how the subconscious mind works.

But not everybody understands how they can use this power of the mind to help themselves accomplish success in about every little thing they do. Some just go through life by depending on the results of their strategies, the majority of which are failures, without attempting to use the power they have.

If you have objectives to accomplish or things that you prefer, you can be victorious in having or attaining whatever it is by understanding how the subconscious mind works then try to use it. But right before anything else, you must be asking: What is the subconscious mind?

First you need to know that the mind is separated into 2: the mindful and the subconscious.

The mindful mind is the part accountable for all ideas that you are presently knowledgeable about. This is the part that's working when you're making choices, reductions, and other thinking procedures including reason and reasoning.

The subconscious, on the other hand, is essentially the part of the human mind that includes an individual's beliefs and routines. These are the ideas that are incorporated into the mind long previously, generally at youth.

Your youth experiences essentially lay the structures for your ideas, beliefs and practices you perform your life. They produce what is in some cases described as 'your map of reality'. What you see, hear, feel and experience throughout the early years is constantly being inscribed on your subconscious mind. All this info is then processed and used to produce your really own external reality.

Let's say for instance, your mother and father continuously told you as a kid that life was a battle and cash was always limited. Repeated sufficient times, this sort of info will enter into your subconscious programs.

As you advance through life this shows will keep playing out time and time again, suggesting that your life experiences will be that befitting to battle and deficiency. Understand on how the subconscious mind works? The good idea nevertheless, is that you can eliminate and re-write the youth programs that are held deep within your subconscious mind.

Below are some easy approaches you can begin using today to gradually reprogram your subconscious so you can start appreciating a lot more success in your life.

1. Incorporate your Goals/Ideas into the Subconscious
When you have an objective for instance, to be a physician, or expert athlete you should imagine yourself being a lot like one, consistently every day. The objective is to integrate the idea that you will, one day, become a physician or expert athlete, into your subconscious mind. Doing this consistently will gradually but undoubtedly change your configured beliefs which will power you on to attaining success with this specific objective.

2. Make Demands to your Subconscious Mind
The subconscious mind does not rest. It continuously works even at sleep. Making demands to the subconscious is done by verifying aloud the important things you want to have, do and be and after that envisioning them right before you go to sleep.
For instance, you want to become an expert speaker, but you hesitate that you do not have the self-confidence and capability to speak in front of hundreds or countless people.
Close your eyes and speak up with feeling "I am a positive, fascinating and motivating speaker", and after that envision yourself abandoning phase in an auditorium of countless people and talking to them with supreme self-confidence and fluency.

Do this each time previous to going to sleep and the power of your subconscious mind will pick up your demand and will gradually and certainly find the methods and means for you to accomplish and understand this objective. How your brain works can be truly effective. The brain doesn't only let you examine things but it can also form your character and beliefs.

But its understanding how the subconscious mind works that is the real key to an effective life. In other words it's the engine which runs your entire life. The top factor to where your fate lies. learn how to use it effectively and you actually can accomplish success without actually needing to try really hard.

Your subconscious mind is the crucial to you attaining every objective and dream you have ever had. When you really find how the subconscious mind works you will then hold the key to open the door to a brand-new and

remarkable life. Extraordinary riches, great success and unrestricted joy are
ensured to be yours.

Chapter 3: Multiple Sclerosis

Meaning of Multiple Sclerosis

Multiple Sclerosis is a persistent health problem of the main nerve system
which has results on the body's defense system.

Individuals that have passed the age of thirty typically develop Multiple
Sclerosis, and there are a lot more ladies than guys experiencing the illness.
More than one million people are impacted by Multiple Sclerosis.

The main nerve system is made from the brain and the spinal column and
without it, the body could not live and believe, since it processes the signals
transferred by the nerve endings that are spread out all over the body and
reacts to them. Multiple Sclerosis impacts this procedure and for that reason
disrupts our capabilities to taste, odor, touch and feels every little thing.

The nerves of the main nerve system are surrounded by membrane called
myelin. This membrane is impacted by Multiple Sclerosis as it makes the
main nerve system attack it by sending out the antibodies and the leukocyte
against it.

Leukocyte and antibodies are cells that have the purpose of battling bacterial
and viral infections. Whenever a hazardous foreign microbe gets in the body
and it begins an infection the main nerve system sends out the antibodies ruin
it. Multiple Sclerosis puzzles the main nerve system and makes it send out
the leukocyte against the myelin. They assault it and after that the nerves
become faulty. In time, Multiple Sclerosis totally blocks the nerve signals and
seriously impacts the senses.

Multiple Sclerosis' causes aren't completely understood. Scientists are still
studying what the reasons for the antibodies attacks are. MC might have a
hereditary cause but this is not exactly sure yet. The signs of Multiple
Sclerosis are really different from one client to another, depending upon what
senses are impacted.

Here is a list of general signs that might appear:
complete or partial short-term loss of vision. Vision usually gets fuzzy or double.

confusion, Tiredness, Weak Point, Lightheadedness, Trembling, abnormal Movement, Balance Loss

Hand or Leg paralysis

Incoherent Speech

These are just a few of the signs, each client presents specific signs since there are a ton of nerve endings in the body and every one can be impacted and shows a very different sign.

Comprehending the Subtypes

Depending upon its patterns of development, along with the strength and frequency of its produced signs, Multiple Sclerosis can be classified in 7 different subtypes.

The very first subtype of Multiple Sclerosis is the relapsing-remitting Multiple Sclerosis (RR MS), the most typical form of the autoimmune condition. According to stats, more than 80 percent of all Multiple Sclerosis cases are of the relapsing-remitting subtype. This subtype is identified by stages of symptomatic remission, followed by stages of regression (defined by unexpected accumulation of signs). The period of the stages of regression and remission differ from a client to another, lasting anywhere from some weeks to some years.

The 2nd subtype of Multiple Sclerosis - primary-progressive Multiple Sclerosis (PP MS) represents around 20 percent of all Multiple Sclerosis cases. The significant qualities of the subtype are progressive development of the illness, with really brief stages of remission. The 3rd Multiple Sclerosis subtype resembles the PP MS subtype and is called secondary-progressive Multiple Sclerosis (SP MS). Clients with primary-progressive Multiple Sclerosis have half chances to ultimately develop secondary-progressive Multiple Sclerosis.

The 4th subtype of Multiple Sclerosis is called progressive-relapsing Multiple Sclerosis (PR MS) and is identified by progressive development with regular stages of symptomatic worsening.

The 5th Multiple Sclerosis subtype alternates between the primary-progressive, secondary-progressive and progressive-relapsing types of the illness.

The 6th Multiple Sclerosis subtype is benign Multiple Sclerosis, defined by a preliminary symptomatic flare which can be followed by sluggish or no development at all.

The seventh and last Multiple Sclerosis subtype is also extremely uncommon. It is called deadly Multiple Sclerosis and includes quick development and extremely extreme signs. This subtype is in a lot of cases fatal.

Typical Signs

The symptomatic spectrum of Multiple Sclerosis can be extremely varied, including different symptoms according to the impacted body areas. Multiple Sclerosis is an inflammatory neural illness, triggering dysfunctions primarily at the level of the main nerve system. Due to the simple fact that Multiple Sclerosis impacts the nerve system, people with this form of neural illness can in time experience signs in the majority of innervated areas of the body.

Multiple Sclerosis includes damage of the worried cells, ruining myelin, a compound that generally covers nerve cells. Myelin has a crucial role in sending anxious impulses throughout the whole body, developing connections between the surrounding worried cells. When the layers of myelin are impacted, anxious impulses travel at decreased speed between nerve cells and the body is not able to sufficiently react to external stimuli.

The signs of Multiple Sclerosis are varied, and they can be viewed in different areas of the body. The majority of clients have embellished signs of Multiple Sclerosis, and they tend to happen in episodes, or "flares". The development of Multiple Sclerosis is unforeseeable, rotating between phases of remission and phases of regression. Many people with Multiple Sclerosis experience periodic, recidivating signs which magnify in the phases of reoccurrence. Thinking about the simple fact that the signs of Multiple Sclerosis are different and at certain phases of the illness unspecific, Multiple Sclerosis can't be detected only upon scientific symptoms. Multiple Sclerosis is generally identified upon lab tests, blood analyses and intricate neural assessments.

Typical, generalized signs of Multiple Sclerosis are: noticeable tiredness, body weakness, feelings of tingling, burning, strong pain, itching and tingling of the muscles, loss of mastery and uncoordinated body language. Other physical signs of Multiple Sclerosis are: reduced vision, loss of movement, shaking, convulsions, tremblings, poor balance, lightheadedness, vertigo. In later phases of the illness, the signs of Multiple Sclerosis can consist of partial paralysis, kidney and intestinal dysfunctions.

Neuropsychological signs of Multiple Sclerosis are psychological confusion; modified, incorrect understandings; poor concentration; short-term amnesia; jeopardized judgment and unforeseeable, unexpected changes of state of mind. A sign of Multiple Sclerosis that frequently takes place in people with this form of neural illness is anxiety. The majority of people impacted by Multiple Sclerosis ultimately become depressed and stay away from any type of interaction with other individuals.

Although a lot of signs of Multiple Sclerosis can be really noticeable at certain phases of the illness, they can be eased through the ways of medical treatment. Medical treatments readily available today have the ability to alleviate the signs of Multiple Sclerosis in the durations of regression and in time they can even help the restoration of myelin, hence assisting clients to recuperate from the illness. It is very important to prompt find the signs of Multiple Sclerosis so as to start the administration of a proper medical treatment right before the illness ends up being serious.

Probable Causes of Multiple Sclerosis

Although the precise causes and threat aspects of Multiple Sclerosis are still unidentified to contemporary medical science, it is really believed that the illness happens on the properties of acquired hereditary dysfunctions and is activated by certain ecological aspects (either direct exposure to substances or infections with infections or germs). In spite of the simple fact that medical researchers have performed fancy research on Multiple Sclerosis over the last couple of years, the precise genes that render people more prone to developing the autoimmune condition and the precise ecological causative representatives have not been recognized yet.

According to current research studies in the field, hereditary elements play a major role in the incident and development of Multiple Sclerosis. Medical researchers notify that Multiple Sclerosis has a noticeable genetic character, the genes that render people vulnerable of developing the condition being transmissible from one generation to another. Current medical research has exposed the simple fact that the twin of an individual detected with Multiple Sclerosis has a 30 percent chance of developing the exact same condition at a particular point in life.

The danger of very first degree loved ones of individuals with Multiple Sclerosis to develop the condition is 50 times higher than that of individuals without any family history of Multiple Sclerosis. Medical researchers are presently working to determine the precise genes that render individuals with a family history of Multiple Sclerosis vulnerable to developing the condition at a particular phase in life.

Medical researchers actually believe that infections with infections are also possible reasons for Multiple Sclerosis. This belief is supported by the unequal geographical circulation of the illness (cases of Multiple Sclerosis are more many in areas of the World faced with routine cases of viral illnesses). In addition, researchers have developed a link between Multiple Sclerosis and viral upsurges. According to the actual results of medical examinations, the general number of Multiple Sclerosis cases increases throughout viral upsurges. In addition, certain infections are extremely comparable to myelin (the protein that is mainly impacted by Multiple Sclerosis), and it is thought that such infections puzzle the body immune system, identifying its antibodies to target the body's healthy afferent neuron covered in myelin rather than the intruding contagious representatives.

The transmittable organisms that are thought to contribute in the event and development of Multiple Sclerosis are herpes infections and Chlamydia pneumoniae germs. The HHV-6 subtype of herpes infection (infection that triggers rosella in kids) has also been recognized to trigger extreme illnesses of the nerve system just like sleeping sickness (brain swelling). Other subtypes of herpes infections like herpes simplex 1 and 2; varicella-zoster infection and cytomegalovirus also have potential of triggering dysfunctions of the nerve system. Chlamydia pneumoniae, an irregular germ that has been related to numerous inflammatory illnesses is also presumed to trigger Multiple Sclerosis. Although medical research continues, indications of infection with Chlamydia pneumoniae have been exposed in the bulk of clients with Multiple Sclerosis.

Other prospective reasons for Multiple Sclerosis are physical injuries (injuries at the level of the spine), in addition to psychological tension (current research studies have exposed that the signs of Multiple Sclerosis are magnified on the facilities of psychological tension).

Requirements for Being Identified with Multiple Sclerosis

Multiple Sclerosis is an inflammatory neural illness which produces a broad symptomatic spectrum. Multiple Sclerosis mainly impacts the main nerve system, disrupting the typical activity of the worried cells. Multiple Sclerosis includes wear and tear of the nerve cells' myelin, a really essential compound that helps with the transference of anxious signals between worried cells. If myelin is impacted, the connections between nerve cells are jeopardized and the body stops working to react quickly to external stimuli.

Multiple Sclerosis can trigger numerous dysfunctions in different areas of the body, triggering a vast array of physical, neural and mental symptoms. The wear and tear of myelin can impact the body's motor functions, triggering trouble walking, loss of mastery, inadequately collaborated relocations, vertigo; sensorial functions, triggering reduced visual skill, transformed understandings of external stimuli; and cognitive functions, triggering poor psychological efficiency, loss of concentration and even amnesia. In many cases, Multiple Sclerosis can even hinder the typical activity of the inner organs, triggering kidney love and conditions of the intestinal system.

Due to the complicated nature of Multiple Sclerosis signs, it is essentially unrealistic to identify the illness relying exclusively on clients' external symptoms. The signs created by neural illnesses have an unspecific character, therefore making the procedure of Multiple Sclerosis medical diagnosis a lot harder. For this reason, Multiple Sclerosis can be properly identified only after carrying out sophisticated physical exams and different lab tests.

Multiple Sclerosis medical diagnosis includes the build-up of different suggestive information through the ways of particular medical treatments and lab analyses. The initial step in the procedure of Multiple Sclerosis medical diagnosis generally includes the evaluation of clients' motor functions. Individuals with this kind of neural illness usually have trouble walking and keeping their balance. Loss of mastery, muscle weakness and inadequately collaborated relocations are also suggestive indications for Multiple Sclerosis medical diagnosis. Additionally, sensorial dysfunctions, like reduced vision, are really typical to people with neural illnesses and a crucial Multiple Sclerosis medical diagnosis requirement includes trying to find indications of internuclear ophthalmoplegia (double, blurred vision).

The procedure of Multiple Sclerosis medical diagnosis typically includes MRI scans and back leak. MRI scans (magnetic resonance imaging) are a crucial step in validating the Multiple Sclerosis medical diagnosis. MRI scans confirm the stability of the nerve system, using magnetic waves for creating images. If MRI scans can often be undetermined in the procedure of Multiple Sclerosis medical diagnosis, back leak is a trustworthy requirement in confirming the presence of neural illness. Through the methods of back leak, medical professionals have the ability to check the state of the spines fluid, looking for proof of swelling at the level of the nerve system.

Neuropsychological tests are also extremely essential in the procedure of Multiple Sclerosis medical diagnosis. The aim of these tests is to find proof of jeopardized psychological efficiency because of damage of myelin. A lot of clients with neural illnesses typically experience poor concentration, reduced judgment and even short-term amnesia and the primary purpose of neuropsychological tests is to expose the presence of these signs. Another essential step in developing the Multiple Sclerosis medical diagnosis includes trying to find indications of anxiety, as more than 80 percent of people impacted by this kind of neural illness ultimately become depressed.

Multiple Sclerosis medical diagnosis is really intricate and needs numerous medical treatments and tests for exposing definitive indications of the illness. The majority of clients are identified with Multiple Sclerosis only if more than 2 particular tests verify the presence of neural dysfunctions.

Types and Treatments

Multiple Sclerosis includes an inflammatory procedure at the level of the main nerve system, leading to the damage of myelin. Myelin is a compound that surrounds the body's worried cells, helping with the transference of worried impulses between nerve cells. If the stability of the anxious cells' myelin is jeopardized, the transference of anxious impulses between nerve cells is worried, triggering serious neural dysfunctions.

Multiple Sclerosis mostly impacts the body's capability to react quickly to external stimuli (sensorial function), reduces the movement of the musculoskeletal system (motor function) and lowers psychological efficiency (cognitive function). People impacted by Multiple Sclerosis can in time experience serious neuropsychological conditions, just like: anxiety, short-term amnesia, jeopardized judgment, mental illness, mania and even dementia. Multiple Sclerosis can also impact the activity of the inner organs, triggering kidney dysfunctions or conditions of the intestinal system.

Multiple Sclerosis can impact the whole activity of the body and people who experience this illness can develop serious physical and neuropsychological conditions. The development of Multiple Sclerosis is periodic and unforeseeable. Individuals impacted by Multiple Sclerosis can experience durations of remission, followed by states of regression. The signs produced by the illness happen in episodes, or flares.

Although the majority of the damage brought on by this kind of neural illness to the organism can be lessened and reversed with the methods of a suitable Multiple Sclerosis treatment, contemporary medication does not hold the remedy for this specific kind of illness. Most of Multiple Sclerosis treatments readily available today are concentrated on extending the durations of remission and on decreasing the period and the strength of symptomatic flares, being not able to totally get rid of the illness.

The most efficient medication used in Multiple Sclerosis treatments is beta interferon. This compound is frequently used in Multiple Sclerosis treatments for assisting in the procedure of myelin restoration. By utilizing beta interferon in Multiple Sclerosis treatments, physicians have the ability to manage the development of the illness and to eliminate the real reasons for its produced neural dysfunctions.

Thinking about the simple fact that the illness also produces muscle weakness, swelling, strong pain and rigidness, most of Multiple Sclerosis treatments consist of nonsteroidal anti-inflammatory drugs, which can help in reducing the signs experienced at the level of the musculoskeletal system. Corticosteroids are also typically used in Multiple Sclerosis treatments, as they can reduce the strength of the physical signs experienced throughout the phases of regression. Multiple Sclerosis treatments typically consist of anticonvulsants, analgesics, moderate sedatives and muscle relaxants in the durations of symptomatic worsening.

If clients develop inner conditions as a result of unsuitable activity of the nerve system, Multiple Sclerosis treatments can also include making use of medications like anticholinergics (drugs that minimize bladder convulsions), urinary system antispasmodics and antidiuretics.

For enhancing psychological efficiency, memory and concentration, Multiple Sclerosis treatments can also consist of Selective Serotonin Reuptake Inhibitors and Central Nerve System Stimulants. These medications have the ability to reduce the generalized state of psychological tiredness particular to people impacted by Multiple Sclerosis. If clients experience serious mental conditions, like anxiety or mental illness, Multiple Sclerosis treatments can also include using anti-depressives and moderate sedatives.

Advantages of Treatment for Multiple Sclerosis

Multiple Sclerosis is an inflammatory neural illness that can produce a vast array of physical and mental signs. Multiple sclerosis includes the wear and tear of myelin, a compound that surrounds the body's anxious cells. Myelin has a really essential role in the transference of worried impulses, and if this compound is impacted, the whole activity of the nerve system is seriously jeopardized.

Although the real reasons for Multiple Sclerosis stay unidentified, there are some hypotheses that present hereditary irregularities as the primary aspects accountable for triggering the illness. Medical researchers actually believe that Multiple Sclerosis takes place on the background of acquired hereditary predispositions, and ecological elements are believed to be triggers of the illness. Some hypotheses also introduce viral infections in this circumstance, though infections with infections do not appear to add to the development of the illness.

Multiple Sclerosis can impact the body on different levels. Most of people with Multiple Sclerosis struggle with dysfunctions of the muscular system, while other ones also develop neuropsychological dysfunctions. Multiple Sclerosis generally creates a large range of signs: body weakness, pronounced tiredness, muscle feeling numb, inadequately collaborated relocations, poor balance. Individuals impacted by Multiple Sclerosis can in time experience reduced visual skill, mindsets of confusion and even short-term amnesia. Individuals with Multiple Sclerosis can also experience anxiety, which prevails in more than 80 percent of clients with the illness.

Although there is no treatment for Multiple Sclerosis, many medical treatments can ease the signs produced by the illness, also stopping their reoccurrence. Nevertheless, most of medications recommended in long-lasting Multiple Sclerosis treatments (beta interferon, corticosteroids) can produce a lot of side-effects, triggering extra damage to the body. Thus, it is best to stay away from following long-lasting treatments with potentially-harmful drugs.

In a lot of cases, Multiple Sclerosis treatments can ameliorate physical signs just as well, without using any drugs. Thinking about the simple fact that the majority of signs produced by the illness are connected to the musculoskeletal system, most of Multiple Sclerosis treatments are concentrated on enhancing muscular movement and tonus through workout. Multiple Sclerosis treatment through workout can help clients restore their strength, coordination and balance, minimizing muscular strong pain, pins and needles and tightness.

Most of Multiple Sclerosis treatments include recuperative workouts and medical gymnastics. Other types of Multiple Sclerosis treatments consist of leisure exercises, just like swimming, running or the practice of different sports. Many people who have followed such Multiple Sclerosis treatments have experienced an amelioration of their physical signs and have enhanced their total health condition. Although medical treatments are needed for many clients, people who follow Multiple Sclerosis treatment really need littler dosages of medications. Integrated with a proper diet plan and a healthy way of life, Multiple Sclerosis treatment through workout can be extremely advantageous.

Tips for an Adjusted Diet plan

A pretty good Multiple Sclerosis diet plan is actually believed to help control and perhaps remove a lot of the signs that come along with the illness. This can help slow the development of the illness. While you should talk to a medical professional for particular tips or standards, there are some standard pointers to a Multiple Sclerosis diet plan.

An vital part of a healthy Multiple Sclerosis diet plan is to get rid of all gluten. In general, you should keep away from eating anything with flour, but you can check bundle components if you are not sure of their content. Numerous diet plans besides the Multiple Sclerosis diet plan do not enable gluten, so this is now quickly found on a lot of plans. Keeping away from wheat s, barley, oats, or rye is another way to cut gluten.

For an effective Multiple Sclerosis diet plan you should also restrict or stay away from animal fats, consisting of dairy items and margarine. Olive oil, sunflower oil, and safflower oil appropriate options for cooking or salads. For great food digestion, you should try to stay away from fried foods in general.

Keep away from highly hydrogenated fats in your Multiple Sclerosis diet plan. Breast meat skinless chicken, seafood, and fish are the best meat choices. Make certain to always entirely eliminate any fat. Try to change the hydrogenated fats you eliminated with unsaturated fats.

Anybody, but particularly those on a Multiple Sclerosis diet plan, should try to totally remove refined sugar. There are tons of much healthier options. Honey, fructose, or natural unsweetened fruit or veggie juices would be ideal for an individual on a Multiple Sclerosis diet plan.

Undoubtedly, any foods you dislike should be cut from your Multiple Sclerosis diet plan. If you are not sure of allergic reactions, try speaking with a medical professional or allergic reaction professional. You might also try getting rid of all of the most typical issue foods from your diet plan, and after 2 weeks bring them back one at a time. If you have a bad response to any food, then you should most likely remove it from your Multiple Sclerosis diet plan.

You should increase the number of fresh veggies and fruits in your Multiple Sclerosis diet plan. Try to always eat newly prepared food when you should prepare it. This will increase the amount of minerals and vitamins your body takes in. This will help to make up for some of the nutrients you lose by cutting certain things from your diet plan. Vitamin supplements might also be advantageous and even essential for your Multiple Sclerosis diet plan, but you should speak with a physician to make certain you take the right vitamins.

Always drink a lot of water in your Multiple Sclerosis diet plan. It is really simple for an individual with Multiple Sclerosis to become dehydrated, so make certain to drink at least 8 big glasses of water every day. As odd as it sounds, this might help to enhance the incontinence that lots of people with Multiple Sclerosis struggle with.

These suggestions for enhancing your Multiple Sclerosis diet plan are meant to help you manage tons of typical issues like tiredness, incontinence, and irregularity. Changing your Multiple Sclerosis diet plan might also help to stay away from making other issues even worse. Lots of these suggestions are included in other diet plans, and even people without unique dietary requirements might take advantage of following these tips.

How It Develops

Multiple Sclerosis is a kind of autoimmune illness that typically triggers permanent disabilities at different levels of the nerve system. At present, Multiple Sclerosis can neither be stopped, nor entirely treated. Nevertheless, the existing treatments are used to decrease the development of the illness, extend the durations of remission, reduce the symptomatic flare-ups and stop the development of more issues. The primary element accountable for the development of Multiple Sclerosis is improper activity of the body immune system.

While the typical body immune system produces antibodies that combat against antigens (foreign contagious representatives), when it comes to

Multiple Sclerosis the body immune system ends up being inefficient and turns against healthy body cells. The jeopardized body immune system can no longer compare healthy, regular cells and antigens, setting off repeated attacks on the body's nerve system and damaging the anxious cells' protective cover called myelin. The damage of myelin (protein that has a series of crucial roles at the level of the nerve system) figures out serious disabilities of the main nerve system and peripheral nerve tissues.

Myelin surrounds the axons, (filaments that are accountable with the transference of electrical impulses amongst afferent neuron) helping with the transference of info between anxious cells. When the myelin cover is damaged, the signals transferred at the level of the nerve system are interrupted, therefore triggering a series of neural signs in clients challenged with this kind of illness. Although in the past medical researchers actually believed that Multiple Sclerosis only includes the damage of myelin, current medical examinations have exposed the simple fact that the axons are also assaulted by the inefficient body immune system.

Axon damage starts in the incipient phases of Multiple Sclerosis and it is thought about to be the primary reason for the irreparable character of the illness. The spontaneous durations of remission experienced by many clients with Multiple Sclerosis are actually believed to take place not as a result of short-term reduced autoimmune reaction, but as a result of emphasized remyelination (fixing of the myelin) at the level of the afferent neuron. Nevertheless, the benefic results of remyelination are later gone beyond by the unwanted actions of the body immune system in the durations of regression. Captivated by the procedure of spontaneous remyelination that takes place in the durations of remission, medical researchers are presently working to promote and improve this procedure at the level of the afferent neuron in clients with Multiple Sclerosis. Additional stimulation of the nerve systems' production of myelin, substantiated with immunosuppressive treatments might supply an effective remedy in the future.

Effects of Myelin damage

Multiple Sclerosis is an inflammatory illness that mostly impacts the brain and spine (the main nerve system of the body - CNS). In later phases of the illness, Multiple Sclerosis can include practically any innervated area of the body (body parts which consist of structures of agglomerated nerve terminations). By impacting the nerve fibers which have the role to transfer signals between the main nerve system and all the innervated organs, Multiple Sclerosis can trigger a wide variety of problems at different levels of the body. When Multiple Sclerosis includes more parts of the body, the created signs considerably differ in regards to type and strength, rendering the procedure of detecting the illness really troublesome.

Although the development of Multiple Sclerosis can be effectively managed and its produced signs can be eased, the already current damage can't be reversed with medical treatments. Therefore, the speed and precision of medical diagnosis play essential roles in stopping the development of more issues and also increase the performance of the particular medication treatments.

All the unwanted impacts produced by Multiple Sclerosis take place because of damage of myelin, a compound that surrounds the cells of the nerve system. The primary role of myelin is to help with the transference of nerve signals at the level of main nerve system and between the CNS and all the other nerves spread out throughout the body. Myelin also has the role to safeguard afferent neuron, forming a finishing that surrounds their surface area. Most of the times, the damage of myelin particular to Multiple Sclerosis occurs quickly and produces a vast array of dysfunctions of the nerve system. The procedure of myelin damage is irreparable and most current medical treatments can only decrease this procedure, being not able to stop it.

Due to the simple fact that Multiple Sclerosis can trigger a plethora of dysfunctions in different areas of the body, the type, strength and period of signs vary from a client to another. Clients with Multiple Sclerosis might experience tingling, tingling or strong pain in the muscles, muscular weakness and tiredness, muscular convulsions, reduced visual skill, blurred and double vision, regular urination, irregularity, reduced sexual function, poor balance, queasiness, short-term amnesia, reduced judgment, poor concentration, and so on. The list of Multiple Sclerosis signs is long and such symptoms might either take place together or individually, depending upon the levels of the nerve system which are impacted by the illness.

Fortunately, is that clients with Multiple Sclerosis who get the sufficient medical treatment can gain back control of their bodies and live active, typical lives. Although they can't reverse the already existing nerve damage nor entirely treat the illness, the majority of Multiple Sclerosis treatments can significantly relieve signs and stop the event of extreme problems.

Medication

Today's treatments for Multiple Sclerosis mainly aim to decrease the development of the illness, stop the development of more problems and reduce the existing signs. At present there is no particular remedy for Multiple Sclerosis and hence no medical treatment can totally get rid of the illness. In addition, the medications used in Multiple Sclerosis treatments can't reverse the nerve damage brought on by Multiple Sclerosis; they can only stop future damage by decreasing the devastating potential of numerous aspects that sustain the illness (Multiple Sclerosis includes an autoimmune reaction of the body, identifying the body immune system to ruin healthy afferent neuron rather than intruding contagious representatives). Nevertheless, clients who get the proper treatment prompt and in the right dosages can live regular, active lives and get control over their signs.

The medications that have shown really effective in managing the development of Multiple Sclerosis and relieving its signs are Avonex, Betaseron and Copaxone. Popular under the name of "ABC drugs", Avonex, Betaseron and Copaxone are thoroughly used to counter signs like tiredness and muscular weakness, symptoms that have been related to Multiple Sclerosis and different other looking like autoimmune conditions. Although Avonex, Betaseron and Copaxone all have distinct qualities, they all have the exact same objective - to minimize the damage brought on by the inefficient body immune system to healthy anxious cells by different natural systems. Administered in the suitable dosage, each unique medication from the classification of "ABC drugs" can lower the frequency and strength of Multiple Sclerosis by approximately a 3rd.

Avonex (Beta-interferon-1a) - This medication is typically used in the treatment of Multiple Sclerosis and is administered under the form of intramuscular injections. Avonex can significantly minimize swelling at the level of the impacted afferent neuron and can decrease the procedure of demyelization (the procedure of myelin damage). Administered to clients in early phases of Multiple Sclerosis, Avonex can stop the incident of problems just like dysfunctions of the motor system (that includes muscles and connective tissues), vertigo, visual and hearing issues, speech issues, memory issues and other comparable cognitive disabilities (happen when different parts of the brain are impacted by Multiple Sclerosis).

Although Avonex can produce side-effects just like fever, chills, muscular pain and strong pain, these signs aren't really extreme and only last for several hours after the injection. The side-effects of Avonex can be managed by utilizing ibuprofen or acetaminophen-based drugs right before or right after each injection.

Betaseron (Beta-interferon-1b) - This drug is also extremely reliable in managing the signs of Multiple Sclerosis and minimizing the dangers of problems. Betaseron is administered under the form of non-painful subcutaneous injections and is well endured by the majority of clients. Periodically, Betaseron can produce side-effects like skin inflammation at the site of injection, moderate fever and tiredness. The drug is the main choice in the treatment of secondary-progressive Multiple Sclerosis, a subtype of the illness defined by steady development.

Copaxone (Glatiramer acetate or Copolymer-1) - Included in the treatment of Multiple Sclerosis, this medication is also extremely effective in relieving signs and stopping the event of problems. The drug is provided under the form of subcutaneous injections. Compared to the formerly defined drugs, Copaxone has really couple of side-effects and is well endured by many clients. Copaxone is thought about to be a safe medication and appropriates for a lot of classifications of clients with Multiple Sclerosis.

Comprehending the Diagnosis

Once an individual has been detected with MS the next question many people ask is "What is my diagnosis with Multiple Sclerosis?" If they have found out about the illness, lots of have heard only the absolute worst case circumstance and expect to only have several years at finest to live. Due the nature of the specific illness the diagnosis for most of clients is that they will live for several years, in a lot of cases their life-span is at worst only very likely to be reduced by several years.

Specifying the Diagnosis of Multiple Sclerosis
The very nature of the illness and the simple fact that it doesn't appear to impact any 2 people in the exact same way can make forecasting diagnosis for Multiple Sclerosis extremely tough. Nevertheless, there are certain aspects that can help physicians identify a short-term diagnosis that can be changed depending upon how quickly the illness advances. To begin with less than 55 of all people detected with MS are understood to have the most serious form of progressive MS.

Of all people detected with Multiple Sclerosis some 10-20% are found to have the benign range which advances so gradually that any development might not even be noticeable. A current research study shows that at least 7 out of every 10 clients who are identified with MS will still live 25 years after they are detected. This is close to the 9 out of 10 people of the exact same age who do not have this illness.

Aspects that can impact a Multiple Sclerosis Diagnosis
There are a lot of aspects that can impact the diagnosis of Multiple Sclerosis. Whether you are a male or a female makes a big difference as the illness has been revealed to reduce the lives of guys by approximately 11 years and ladies by only 6 years. Most of the times when you are identified with the benign kind of MS your chances of ending up being handicapped are fairly little. Those who do experience some level of special needs in the very first 5 years are very likely to see a 75% boost in the special needs by the time 10-15 years has passed.

There are actions you can require enhancing your Multiple Sclerosis diagnosis beyond the drug treatments that your medical professional is very likely to put you on. While the illness is very likely to make you become quickly tired out, routine of workout has been found to help decrease the development and minimize the effect of any worsenings you may experience. Even if your signs consist of partial paralysis you can still continue to work out.

Eating a well-balanced diet plan will have a major effect your diagnosis. Removing overtly processed foods and red meats can help in reducing the amount of swelling in your body. Stay with leafy green veggies and fruit in addition to lean meats and foods that are high in Omega 3 fats has been shown to have a major influence on regressions and just how long you can expect to live conveniently.

Spasticity

Among the most typical indications of Multiple Sclerosis is spasticity, which it the most usually referred to as unmanageable muscle convulsions or contractions that do not work in sync with the other muscles in a limb. This specific issue can also manifest itself as muscles that are stiff and withstand hidden muscle movement. It can also trigger the MS client to feel a particular amount of real pain in their joints and while this sign can manifest itself in any of the client's limbs it happens mainly in the legs.

What Triggers Multiple Sclerosis Spasticity?

As Multiple Sclerosis triggers damage to the myelin sheath that surrounds both the brain and the spine it has a direct impact on the transfer of info from the nerves to the brain and back again. In many cases these signals move far too gradually to be efficient, in other ones the signals get rushed as they travel.

Great motor abilities are something we develop as we grow from an infant into an adult and this needs the brain to be able to communicate efficiently with every muscle in our body. With Multiple Sclerosis spasticity, the brain is no longer able to communicate precisely and efficiently with certain muscles and the outcome combined messages trigger the muscles to spasm or alternatively secure ending up being unmanageable.

These episodes can be induced without external stimulation or they can also be brought on by something as easy as being excessively worn out or wearing outfits that are too tight. Depending upon the amount of damage and the area of the MS sores this Multiple Sclerosis spasticity can also become an irreversible part of the client's life.

Are there Treatments for Spasticity?
The most essential thing to keep in mind is that if you do not look for treatment for this Multiple Sclerosis spasticity you could wind up with even more serious issues just like completely frozen joints that will stagnate

leaving you handicapped. Luckily there are some popular and effective treatments that can help eliminate the convulsions and tight muscles that can be really unpleasant.

You should begin by talking with a physio therapist who deals with other MS clients, that way they will already have an idea of what your requirements are. Since each client is different he must begin by assessing the intensity of your spasticity. This is the only way he can create a suggestion as the kind of physical treatment you are going to really need in addition to any medications you should be using.

He will also create a workout routine that is created to keep the muscles as strong and under control as possible. At the exact same time the best thing you can do for your Multiple Sclerosis spasticity is to begin a day-to-day routine of extending and works out to help ease the spasticity and keep it under control. While there is no remedy for the spasticity you can at least learn how to keep it down to a minimum so that you can enjoy your life.

Supplements

Throughout the years, doctor and clients alike have found lots of efficient Multiple Sclerosis supplements. The majority of people that develop this condition are put on medication treatment. The purpose and intent of prescription drugs when used in combination with Multiple Sclerosis is to slow the development of the illness itself, and to relieve the signs that are frequently experienced with Multiple Sclerosis.

Prescriptions might come in the form of tablets, tablets, pills, liquids, and tons of even can be found in the form of a shot that should be administered sometimes weekly. Lots of find that these medications are costly, inefficient, and tons of are bothered by the adverse effects connected with them.

For this reason, Multiple Sclerosis supplements have gotten in appeal. Here, you will learn more about some of the most well-known supplements readily available to the MS client and the advantages related to those supplements.

The Advantages of Taking Supplements
If you are struggling with Multiple Sclerosis, it is very important to

comprehend that there are tons of advantages connected with taking supplements. Not all physicians will motivate using alternative types of treatment for this progressive illness, but it is necessary to speak with a doctor previous to taking any kind of supplement.

While consulting with your medical professional, you might want to present some truths referring to the advantages related to the supplements that you have an interest in. The following represents some of the most typical advantages related to natural supplements:

Tons of Multiple Sclerosis clients have a challenging time when it concerns the body soaking up nutrients from the foodstuff that they take in. If you take the right supplements, your body might have the ability to withdraw the nutrients that it needs to work properly.

If you experience MS, it is vital to comprehend that your body immune system doesn't respond as it must to secure you. As a matter of simple fact, it acts in the opposite way. It actually assaults you. If you take supplements that concentrate on the resistance, this might stop to happen.

Regrettably, swelling is a typical sign of Multiple Sclerosis. A lot of physicians will recommend medications that will lower swelling in the body, but a lot of these might eat at the lining of the stomach and trigger intestinal issues just like ulcers and irritable bowel syndrome. There are certain supplements that will actually work to decrease swelling naturally and with no awkward adverse effects or possible threats.

Among the most typical grievances related to Multiple Sclerosis is reduced energy levels. Lots of supplements will actually supply you with the natural increase that you really need to make it through every day.

The Very Best Supplements
There are lots of Multiple Sclerosis supplements. It is very important to only choose those that help in getting rid of the signs that you find to be awkward. It has been developed by physician that those with MS should take magnesium. It is also essential to have a ton of calcium and even Vitamin D in the body.

Fish oil supplements, night primrose, zinc, copper, the B vitamins, and copper are also rather useful. If you are uncertain of what supplements will benefit you the most, you might have an interest in buying item which contains several vitamins and several minerals.

How to Stop Regressions

For those who have Multiple Sclerosis, a regression or worsening can be among the most aggravating parts of the illness. You might be going along your merry way and after that a regression can happen relatively out of the blue. For the client who is the extremely earliest phases of MS a regression might only happen every couple of months or perhaps years and pass without barely being discovered, though as the illness development the regressions will happen more regularly.

What is a Multiple Sclerosis Regression?

The scientific description of a Multiple Sclerosis regression is a "medically substantial event, simply put an occasion that has apparent signs that can be seen or felt. These regressions are triggered thy sores that happen as a direct outcome of MS on either the client's brain or their spine. It can either be a totally brand-new sign or a worsening of one that you have already experienced. These regressions are also called worsenings, flare or attacks.

The reasons for a regression are normally swellings that happen as outcome of your body immune system assaulting the myelin layer that secures the nerves in your spine and brain. When the attack by the body's immune cells it forms a sore, which is a region of extreme swelling in the location that is under attack. This triggers damage to the location and can decrease or stop the transference of signals from one nerve to another. These lost signals are the origin of the worsenings.

Can I Stop a Multiple Sclerosis Regression?
While a Multiple Sclerosis regression is all part of the illness, there are strategies you can use to minimize the number of regressions you are very likely to have and the frequency with which they take place. A lot of doctors will tell you that the only way to stop a regression is with a consistent program of medications used in illness customizing treatment. There are treatments that have been shown to work and minimize or remove the number of regressions you might have considerably over some years.

Current research is finding that by customizing your way of life and changing the way you eat, it is possible to decrease or get rid of the rate of Multiple Sclerosis regression incidents you are very likely to experience. By eating a diet plan that is wealthy in the foods understood to minimize swelling like kale, lettuce and tons of fruits you can make a major change in how your MS impacts your body. Lots of people now say that by making the essential dietary changes they have been regression totally free for several years.

Tips to Cope with It

Many people start in shock when they are told by their medical professional that they have been identified with MS. The idea of dealing with Multiple Sclerosis can be frightening, particularly to those only know that it is an incurable degenerative illness. While learning to cope with this illness is definitely going to be a fundamental part of your life, there is so much more that you can do to help make things a lot simpler for yourself and to ensure that you manage the illness rather than letting it manage you.

Education
Listening to what your physician needs to outline MS is only a little portion of what you really need to know to make dealing with Multiple Sclerosis. Once you get home and have a good chance to let the truth embedded in, you have 2 choices each of which will lead you in totally different directions. You can sit and let the illness take control of and destroy your life or you can take the bull by the horns and learn every little thing you can about the illness and what you can do to conquer it for the rest of your life.

Thanks to the Web there is a wealth of info on every stage of MS from what researchers believe might be the reason for it to the current research into treatments and medications that are developed to help clients handle it. You can never ever learn way too much and the info is continuously changing as more research is being performed. Use the Web as one of finest resources of info on Multiple Sclerosis.

Eat Well and Workout
Among a lot of frequently advised changes that people dealing with Multiple Sclerosis acknowledge to be the key to remaining in remission and keeping their signs under control is eating a healthy diet plan and working out

frequently. We have all been taught throughout the years how essential it is to eat well and look after our bodies, for the person who has been identified with MS this is more important than ever as correct food and workout can make an incredible distinction.

There have been clients that have reported making significant changes in the choices of foods that they take in has "treated" their MS, while there is no real remedy for Multiple Sclerosis the "remedy" they are speaking about is living totally sign totally free for months and sometimes years. Diet plans that are high in leafy green veggie like cabbage and lettuce in addition to lots of fruits can make a major distinction in the quality of your life. You should also stay with lean meats and lots of fish as it is high in necessary fats

Dealing with Multiple Sclerosis is going to present its share of difficulties over the period of your life. For those who make the choice to learn as much as they can about the illness and make the essential way of life changes it is still possible to lead a really satisfying and long life.

Mental Modification to Multiple Sclerosis

There are at least 5 significant elements of mental change to the illnesses, which are the ones right below.

1. The character of the client
The very first element of mental modification to Multiple Sclerosis is the character of the client. Some clients adjust rapidly to brand-new life whereas other ones are caught in the phase of shock and continue to be depressed for a very long time after the medical diagnosis.

2. The quality of family assistance
The 2nd element of mental modification to Multiple Sclerosis is the quality of assistance readily available to the client within his family. All stakeholders should have an idea about the family characteristics in the past, throughout and after medical diagnosis. They should ask the following questions: Does the client have a life together? What type of relationship the client has with his close family members (kids, partner, and extended family)? The answers to these questions are necessary as the mental suffering of a client might arise from stress within his family (rejection, preconception, exemption,

indifference). Usually a mental maltreatment develops between the client and his family members; they feel not able to bear the everyday development of the illness.

3. The abilities of social openness
The abilities of social openness are the 3rd element of mental modification to Multiple Sclerosis. They in simple fact represent how the client has the ability to look for assistance and psychological peace in his environments specifically his friends and family. It helps the client feel supported in the dissatisfied moment. Continuing his/her job helps the client cope up with the brand-new truths related to the illness since continuing work raises the spirit of the client and fills him with the gut feeling of performance.

4. The quality of the relationship with the medical professional
The quality of the relationship of the client with the physicians (in the broadest sense, which also consists of paramedical workers also) plays as a consider mental change to Multiple Sclerosis. The client has a high level of reliance on his physician for mental assistance in addition to for the management of the illness

5. The illness.
The illness and its diagnosis play an important role in the mental modification of clients with Multiple Sclerosis. If the illness advances gradually, the client gets accustomed to his recently obtained specials needs slowly but if the illness has a fast development, the client cannot change and his life is jeopardized both physically and mentally.

These aspects play an important role in the lifestyle of the client with Multiple Sclerosis. Certainly the most essential aspect is the character of the client who can change with the development of the illness as it advances.

The Lifestyle

Multiple Sclerosis (MS) has a significant influence on lifestyle of clients and might cause a depressive syndrome that is uttered usually by instability, concern, frustration, or uneasiness.

Lifestyle includes 3 primary regions: physical, mental and social. These 3 regions are highly interlinked, social incorporation is typically depending on the physical and mental effect of the illness.

Multiple Sclerosis impacts life at all levels: family, social relations, psychological life, expert life, pastimes and monetary stability. The changing nature and unpredictability of the illness impedes tons of clients in the awareness of a life oriented to the future. It appears that, when given the right tools, people with MS manage to make a location for the illness in their life and to live a significant life with the assistance of their really loved ones.

Multiple Sclerosis is a major reason for neural impairment in young people and usually results in a loss of work several years after medical diagnosis, the typical age of life where work is usually thought about not only essential to provide for his requirements, but also an effective aspect of social incorporation. The illness appears, additionally, to be a barrier to access to big promotion or training.

The rate of absence triggered by MS is on typical 1 month every year and only somewhat higher than for general illnesses. Multiple Sclerosis clients do not have a higher danger of mishaps at work. The 2 significant elements that trigger work interruptions are tiredness and physical conditions. In general they have a strong desire to keep their jobs. Initially they are scared of losing their position and reveal stress and anxiety both at relational and expert level. But after some years of experience, they really appreciate their employability as really positive. They feel more welcome at work and in the house, their complacency considerably enhances, and their vigor increases significantly.

Almost half of the Multiple Sclerosis clients keep the capability to work after they have stopped their occupational activity. Tiredness and cognitive problems are typically pointed out by clients as elements to clarify their work blockage. In the capability to preserve work, individual characteristics, the positive face of illness, ecological aspects like monetary circumstances and family should be considered.

In regard to independent living and everyday travel plans, the rehab of clients of Multiple Sclerosis is always connected to the intensity of disabilities and impairments. The pursuit of a profession is definitely a crucial part of the lifestyle. For this reason, the value of offering people with Multiple Sclerosis the info and assistance in picking the suitable kind of job and work environment.

People with Multiple Sclerosis can live a regular life offered they are supported by their family, good friends, coworkers, healthcare specialists and rehab companies.

Changes with Aging When You Have Multiple Sclerosis

Multiple Sclerosis - a lot of us have already become aware of it, tons of might have watched somebody close struggling with it and I know lots of us are going through it. Whatever our phase is, let's discuss the very first thing very first - what is Multiple Sclerosis? I know, the 2nd question that will pop into your head is - does this one lower our life span like lots of other illnesses? Is there any remedy and if not, could the signs be lessened so that the client could lead a typical life? Might be now you are thinking how I am selecting the right questions to ask. Among my really close associates is dealing with it and when he was very first identified with it, these were the specific questions that strike me.

Aging with Multiple Sclerosis: Physical Changes
Multiple Sclerosis can be thought about an autoimmune condition where the body's body immune system rather than protecting ourselves, begins working against it. In this case, our own body's body immune system assaults the myelin of main nerve system which will cause disability in movement, weakness, blurred vision, vertigo and even paralysis depending upon the intensity of damage.

Multiple Sclerosis and aging are linked. It's not like that you will age right before your time but the age associated issues will appear faster in these clients. It was found that clients having Multiple Sclerosis are in a high danger of developing urinary system infections, cellulitis which is a skin infection triggered by germs and also septicemia which is also called blood poisoning condition where the bacterial infection enters the blood stream, with aging. So, do not forget to watch on them.

Additionally, with aging the possibility of ending up being handicapped will highly increase. Now, the question is how to manage it? In the earlier phase, when the gut feeling of weakness in the leg begins, orthotics which could be used inside shoes could give a genuine help to the foot muscles from getting stiff. In spite of the, climbing upstairs, walking could be frustrating with a weaker leg and don't you stress. 'Ankle foot brace' could help you there. These braces work by supporting ankles when the foot muscles get weak so that you can walk and get up stairs with more ease.

What happens if one leg is more powerful than the other? Yes. We have got resolution for that one too. Take a walking cane on more powerful side and move the body weight to that side so that walking or moving would get much easier. If the damage is substantial in both legs then walkers could be a pretty good choice as it supplies assistance for both of your legs. If you want to have more flexibility, then I believe wheelchairs or power scooters could be the right choice for you.

Changes in cognitive function with aging:
Apart from this physical concern, 65% of Multiple Sclerosis clients struggles with cognitive problems like not able to take note or concentrate, gets sluggish in preparation, info processing and last but not the least loss of memory. Clearly these signs would become worse with aging. Do not believe yourself powerless here. The truth is lots of us could not keep in mind a lot of crucial things. So, it's finest to write in note pads or in computer systems, phones and let the electronic devices do the recalling.

Mental changes with aging:
Now let's get more concerned about the mental concerns. Older Multiple Sclerosis clients experience psychological illness primarily and still do not feel to go to a psychiatrist. Neglecting anxiety, stress and anxiety, tension would be a bad choice to combat this fight. Therapy, occupational treatment could bring a favorable change into your life to help you go through this.

The most frightening feature of aging in Multiple Sclerosis clients is, a time will come when the family will begin seeing the client as a problem as a result of his physical and psychological impairment. I actually found it paradoxical that when the clients needed us most, we want to turn them away.

No, do not get frightened, get prepared. You really need to manage things in a way so that you could do your tasks quickly. And do not forget, you are the fighter here. Don't you ever forfeit, choose therapy, accompany people having exact same issues like you, take aid of a nurse or doctor, take down every little thing so that you do not forget, use assistive gadgets that could help you with movement concerns. See, life is not that challenging. Be strong, be determined, you aren't alone in this battle; we are all here to help you.

Things You Can Do

There are a lot of Multiple Sclerosis workouts that might carried out that are used to help in reinforcing the body and enhancing the client's variety of movement. MS is thought about to be a neural based condition that straight impacts the main nerve system. The main nerve system consists of both the brain and the spine.

This specific system of the body comprises the communication network of the whole body. A lot of people will ultimately experience impairment as the illness advances, but there are some that do not suffer to this degree. People that experience MS ought to develop an interest in workout as it could be the exercise that enhances their health.

Standard Performance
When investigating Multiple Sclerosis workouts, it is necessary to recognize that MS will lead to some degree of loss as far as the body's standard level of performance is concerned. A lot of people have the ability to move from one place to another with ease.

This kind of job generally doesn't take much idea or focused effort. When an individual experiences Multiple Sclerosis, though, easy motions do need both idea and focused effort.

This means that when you perform workouts to build and reinforce the body so that you might keep a high level of self-reliance, you need to do it with care. If you struggle to use care, it is possible to experience physical injuries.

Posture
When carrying out Multiple Sclerosis workouts, it is very important to make sure that you have posture that is thought about to be positive and efficient. Posture, eventually, is the ways in which we hold our body. By making sure that your posture is suitable, you will have the ability to perform a lot of motions with ease.

The right posture will also enable you to experience an ideal exercise that will prove to benefit you in the long run. If you want to experience motions with ease, you need to begin by putting your body in the right position. The right position, naturally, is the right form as it associates with posture.

A lot of that is identified with this condition will enable their gravity center to drop which leads to a modification of posture. Naturally, this will lead to a restricted variety of movement. Sit, stand, and rest with the right posture. You will ultimately see the positive effect it has on your motions.

Selecting Workouts
You might take part in almost any kind of workout that you like when it pertains to Multiple Sclerosis workouts. It is necessary to go over the kinds of motions that you should be carrying out based upon the signs that you are experiencing. It might also be a very good idea to make sure that you aren't alone when you begin working out.

Chapter 4: Memory Strategies

While memory strategies aren't a brand-new thing, the grasp of human memory has always been complex. Human Memory is just one of the most essential things in human knowledge.

Memory is not intelligence, the power of the mind to procedure and subtract is credited to intelligence, but we do know that memory does have some part in helping an effective mind. All clinical disciplines are directed by lots of guidelines and formulas, without memory even the most effective mind would get lost in returning to the exact same standard ideas over and over again. Comprehending is also connected to memory; it is an easy simple fact that once you comprehend some idea or idea you stand a much better chance of remembering it.

All human entities have a minimal capability for memory, there are some uncommon cases of sensational memory capabilities, but the majority of people do not take pleasure in that unusual gift. With our minimal capability people have created tons of types of communication to help us keep in mind ideas and ideas, even centuries old. It not only ideas and ideas that we can enable memory of, it is emotions and feelings, and certain moment in our lives you treasure. Come up with checking out the memories of a historian that resided in the Roman Empire time, offering you know what life was at that time you can comprehend nearly every element of his life.

Although memory is not Intelligence, memory methods train the mind and practice its capability. Memory methods works out increase brain power and is pushing the brain to process what it keeps in mind.

If you just learned an individual's name, imagine relating to how that person will be vital to you in the future, where you are possible to see them consequently, and anything you view about them. Other great reminiscence training includes telling yourself why you wish for keep in mind something, and how you will remember it. Clearly seeing the importance of recalling will promote the brain to hold the name, and the additional links in the brain (where you expect to see the person next, for instance) stick the name a lot more securely in your memory.

The most basic memory exercise to start telling yourself to remember. If you just erudite an individual's name, for instance, notify yourself, "remember that". This suggests the unconscious mind to grade this effort higher in significance.

One memory method goes back to the old Romans, when preparing to make a speech, the roman orator would walk around his garden and associate different parts of the speech to different parts of the garden by positioning parts of the speech at different areas picked right across the garden. A memory strategy that used images, or area is at some point best for people giving speeches, they can use this memory strategy while giving the speech to "walk" themselves around a location they recognize with and keep in mind all the part of the speech. All depends upon images, the more fantastic images you keep in mind, the less chances of forgetting.

A memory method we can try a figured out area like a garden, your office, your home or other places you know all right. Starts by beginning walking around the home and choose 10 spots you will want to put something or associate a memory to. Remember them in your mind in some specific order and hierarchy. Now when you want to keep in mind a list of things, relate them to any of the locations/objects of your office or home. Do this with psychological images and even sounds, always in an absurd way. Now, when you want to remember your list of things, you will just need to walk through your home and every little thing will be clear in your mind.

Better memory begins that moment you comprehend the memory method but does not end till you practice the brand-new memory strategies over and over again. All the best enhancing your memory.

Getting Ahead
Memory methods are extremely basic and can be used to enhance your mind and your life. learn how to boost your mind to impress your good friends or your boss for that pay raise.

Imagine having the ability to remember your grocery list easily, without rote memorization. The human mind is complicated, and with understanding and some memory strategies you will find that knowledge is instilled in your mind, and remembering it will be a breeze.

The Connection Strategy
The connection method produces meaning or a link to an occasion or simple fact that you know, therefore enabling you to remember it quickly. A benefit of the memory strategy is that it utilizes typical info that you know and hence makes it not likely for you to forget the info once the meaning has been connected. For instance, it is simpler to remember an address of 2612 Memory Walk, by connecting it to Boxing Day, which falls on the 26th December.

Mind Mapping
A similarly simple and powerful strategy for training your mind is through mind mapping, which is based upon how we believe and remember info. This memory method uses your whole brain by connecting ideas and procedures. By requiring you to put down on paper your ideas, it requires you to focus your full attention to the info. The use of visuals through colors and images also strengthens memory.

Repeating
This is an easy method typically used to bear in mind something by focusing your whole attention on it. Making use of repeating entrenches the info in

your long term memory. By doing so, you have the ability to keep away from the typical error many individuals make - forgetting things since they did not remember them in the very first spot.

Mnemonics

Mnemonics are a type of memory tool that trains your whole mind to shop and recover info through making use of association. Language is a crucial element of remembering info, and mnemonics in the form of rhymes or familiar trigger words can act as resources to your mind. You can connect the main points or info that you really need to bear in mind in a story, or through making use of acronyms. An example would be Roy of York Delivered fruitless, an acronym for the colors of the rainbow - Red, Orange, Yellow, Green, Blue, Indigo and Violet.

Easy everyday activities like reading is also a great way to enhance your memory by exercising your mind. By learning and using any of the methods above, you will quickly find yourself able to count on your mind more than ever. The capability of our memory is practically unrestricted, and by matching brand-new info to things already in our memory, you will have the ability to train your mind into being a reputable shop of information.

Memory Chunking

Not all people are alike. Some people just are better than the other. This is partially real as whatever it is that you do not have, you can enhance it. All you need to do is to really believe in yourself and do some research on how to enhance yourself. Like for instance, if you have poor memory, you could try looking for methods to make it better. Yes, every little thing is upgradable. Whatever can be enhanced though not as quick as you imagined it to be but it would be a progressive procedure. The bottom line is you could do it. It is possible.

Like earlier pointed out, every little thing can be enhanced. And now, we will concentrate on one element, the memory. Nearly all people surviving on the world is experiencing having issues with recalling things. Do not stress; there are no worms that eat the brain away. It's just a matter of incorrect use of the brain. Not truly that inappropriate but more like inefficient memorizations abilities. Now, if you know these abilities and strategies, you would certainly keep in mind and remember things more effectively that you had previously. These are easy techniques that enable you to optimize your memorization and remembering abilities.

There are a ton of methods and technique readily available for you to make use of to make things far more effective. Consider circumstances the chunking mnemonic memory strategy It is a method to make certain that you would quickly keep in mind numbers, but you could certainly use this on other things too. Put it that way, chunking is organizing down numbers in workable portions to bear in mind it simpler. Just like when you are practicing and attempting to play a guitar solo. You do not copy it as an entire, you divide it into little portions and bits to make the procedure a lot easier to remember.

There are also other kinds of memory strategies that you could use and use in your life to make it much easier for you to remember things. Keep in mind, a pretty good memory could help you become a much better person. Individuals would believe highly of you and you will be a lot more credible. This would also mean that you would also be a much better person when you are at work. Some people are branded careless simply because their poor memory prohibits them to remind them of the obligation that was designated to them. The outcome; say goodbye to duty and people would trust you the least.

So if you just feel like you are having trouble with your memory, I suggest that you follow these memory strategies, it would do you great. And keep in mind, there is absolutely nothing really wrong with you; it is just a matter of how you are going to keep in mind stuff. Using your mind right to remember things is certainly a lot more reliable than anything else. This would absolutely enhance your self - self-confidence, enhance your profession and enhance your relationship with other individuals whether at work, at school or in your home. Try it, you will not regret it.

The Area Memory Strategy can be a reliable tool to help you remember tons of unassociated products. The Area Memory Strategy links the unassociated ideas we want to keep in mind by utilizing remarkable areas to repair the truths or ideas in our memory in a spatial relationship. This strategy is specifically helpful since you can remember any products in precise order.

We know from current hemispheric brain research that our brains serve as computer system file folders, slotting freshly learned info in the exact same file as already-learned info that fits within that exact same file. This method links ideas or products together, just like our brain file folders do. If we put in the time to organize brand-new info in exact same way as our brains, we can enhance our retention of that info.

Background

The age-old Greek orators like Socrates used a unique memory technique that handles familiar item areas. The Greeks would come up with taking a trip of their own houses, starting in the entrances. For each room of the home, they would imagine a keyword of what they were attempting to bear in mind on or beside a unique item in that room. Linking the unidentified (keywords) to the understood (the layout of your home) helps put the keywords into your long term memory.

Directions
Image the layout of your home or apartment or condo. Envision a clockwise walk throughout your home, starting in the entranceway. For each room, image the keyword, or concrete thing, on or beside a specifically remarkable item in that room. Alternative concrete things for any keywords that are too abstract to keep in mind well. For instance, replacing the concrete "bulging bicep" for the abstract strength would be a lot more unforgettable object to image in your dining-room.

Example
Let's say you want to remember the "Preamble to the Constitution."

" We the people of the United States, so as to form a more flawless union, establish justice, make sure domestic harmony, provide for the typical defense, promote the general well-being and protect the true blessings of liberty to ourselves and our posterity do ordain and establish this Constitution for the United States of America."

Keyword remembered in order will help trigger your memory. The keywords aren't always the most essential words. They are the words that will best trigger your memory of the following line(s). In the "Preamble to the Constitution," the keywords may consist of the following: people, in order, justice, make sure, defense, general, true blessings, ordain, for

Using the place method, you may imagine your whole family, connecting arms together, in the entranceway of your home (people). Next, image a playing card royal flush (A, K, Q, J, 10) in order on the sofa in your living-room (in order). Then, image an intense blue law book on the table in your dining-room (justice). Now, image a can of Ensure ® dietary supplement on top of the fridge in your cooking area (make sure). After this, image a white picket fence surrounding the beanbag chair in your living room (defense).

Then, image a GI-Joe ® general saluting you on top of the thermostat in the corridor (general). Next, image yourself sneezing and after that saying "God bless me" on top of the yellow desk in the front bed room (true blessings). After this, image a waiter asking, "May I take your order?" while standing on top of the cabinet in the center bed room (ordain). Finally, image a fluorescent orange "4" on the locked door of the back bedroom (for).

Now timely yourself to bear in mind each simple fact by purposely visualizing the products in each room. Close your eyes, if it helps. Practice walking through your apartment or condo or home and visualizing the specific area of each product to put them into your long-lasting memory.

Got them? The images will stick to you for as long as you really need them. A little wedding rehearsal will keep what you are attempting to remember remain in your memory banks.

Remembering using the Place Memory Method will allow you to keep the memory of a lot of relatively unassociated products.

Example
Let's say you want to remember the "Preamble to the Constitution."

" We the people of the United States, so as to form a more flawless union, establish justice, make sure domestic harmony, provide for the typical defense, promote the general well-being and protect the true blessings of liberty to ourselves and our posterity do ordain and establish this Constitution for the United States of America."

Keyword remembered in order will help trigger your memory. The keywords aren't always the most crucial words. They are the words that will best trigger your memory of the following line(s). In the "Preamble to the Constitution," the keywords may consist of the following: people, in order, justice, make sure, defense, general, true blessings, ordain, for

Using the area technique, you may envision your whole family, connecting arms together, in the entranceway of your home (people). Next, image a playing card royal flush (A, K, Q, J, 10) in order on the sofa in your living-room (in order). Then, image an intense blue law book on the table in your dining-room (justice). Now, image a can of Ensure ® dietary supplement on top of the fridge in your kitchen area (guarantee). After this, image a white picket fence surrounding the beanbag chair in your living room (defense).

Then, image a GI-Joe ® general saluting you on top of the thermostat in the corridor (general). Next, image yourself sneezing and after that saying "God bless me" on top of the yellow desk in the front bed room (true blessings). After this, image a waiter asking, "May I take your order?" while standing on top of the cabinet in the center bed room (ordain). Finally, image a fluorescent orange "4" on the locked door of the back bedroom (for).

Now timely yourself to bear in mind each simple fact by knowingly envisioning the products in each room. Close your eyes, if it helps. Practice walking through your apartment or condo or home and imagining the specific area of each product to put them into your long-lasting memory.

Got them? The images will stick to you for as long as you really need them. A little wedding rehearsal will keep what you are attempting to remember remain in your memory banks.

Remembering using the Place Memory Strategy will allow you to keep the memory of tons of relatively unassociated products.

Connecting

There are some great memory enhancement methods you can learn. Methods that will help in turning numbers into words, remembering names and recalling wish list. Let's talk about how to remember a list of grocery products. We will use 4 products only but you will see the size of the list doesn't matter.

What we do in memory methods is to take something we already know and associate it with something we want to keep in mind. So we link the 2 together or connect them together. We can use what is called the "Roman Room" to connect products together so we can bring them up in our mind in the future.

The reason this works is since there are certain things you will not forget. You know where you live. You know how your home looks and what spaces there are. Presume that you are going to purchase the following products from the shop:

Bananas
Soap
Bread
Paper Towels

Choose any room in your home or condo. Now we will associate the products in the list with something in the room you choose. Envision you walk into your living-room and this is what you see:

Schedule Rack
Table
television
Sofa
These are the very first 4 things you see in series when you enter your living-room. Take each product you want to keep in mind on your wish list and position them with among the products in your living-room or change the product in your room with one from the list.

This is what you may see in your mind:
You walk into your living-room and Bananas are shooting out of your Book Rack. Some Bananas fall onto your Table and are skating on top of Soap. A bar of Soap moves off the Table and approaches the television, but the television is not there. Instead there is a huge loaf of Bread. The huge Bread

eats the Soap but tosses it up all over your Sofa. Out of your Sofa come arms and they are holding Paper Towels and it begins to clean up the mess on itself with the Paper Towels.

We have 2 kinds of memory: the short-term and the long-lasting memory. You can come up with them as 2 doors with the very first one resulting in a little waiting room; and the 2nd door into a large storeroom.

Waiting spaces are spots where people stay temporarily, and storeroom are more long-term. For that reason, anything that goes inside the very first door, but not into the 2nd door, will be lost in the frustrating flow of info that is all around us, making memorization tough.

To stop this are 5 easy memory strategies that will help sharpen your mind and push info from the waiting room to the more long-term, long-lasting storeroom:

1. Concentrate.
Pay more attention to the information that you get so that you can absorb the info better and much faster. Focus your attention while processing realities and figures so that you can take in as much as you can.

2. Make a connection between the brand-new information with something you already know.
The procedure of association is really effective. Use it to link what you want to keep in mind to something you already know or feel deeply about. You can even link it to something completely unassociated.

For instance: say you are asked to purchase diapers on your way home from work. You might link this errand to 'children' or 'stroller.' After 4 hours, you're driving home and see a child being walked by lady crossing the street. You mind will associate the child or the stroller with diapers, which will activate you to keep in mind to purchase the diapers.

3. Repeating.
Tunes and business jingles are simple to remember since they are repeated over and over on the radio and tv. Repeat the info inside your mind again and again. Come up with repeating as overcrowding the waiting room to the point where there is no other spot for the info to go but into long term storage.

4. Organize.
Think of your bed room for a 2nd. When it is unpleasant, it is unrealistic to find anything under all that mess. But when your room is tidy and organized, it's a breeze to find products.

This works the exact same way with your mind.
You not only really need to push memory into storage, but you really need to organize the storeroom well so you can find and remember the info as rapidly and effectively as possible.

So whether you really need to bear in mind lists, realities, or complex ideas, find an approach of organizing information that makes it simple for you to remember and obtain info rapidly.

5. Practice Recalling.
When people come up with memory, they believe strictly about remembering and pushing info into storage. Nevertheless, a fundamental part of memory is about remembering, which means having the ability to obtain all that info from storage. So if you want to truly sharpen memory, learn to practice remembering info you want to remember.

You can practice remembering by remembering something and resting your mind for 5-15 minutes. Then try to recite what you remembered.

If you achieve success, do these steps 3 to 4 more times; each time giving yourself a longer break in between? You may take a bath or check out a book right before returning to remember what you remembered.

If you are still able to keep in mind the information after 3 times, this means the information is living in the part of the brain where it will likely stay long-lasting and where it will be quickly available.

If you struggle at properly reciting the first time around, do not stress. It is alright to flop the very first couple of times. Just routinely use this easy memory strategy whenever you really need to impress a believed in your mind.

These are the pain-free and simple memory methods to help you enhance your memory. Carrying out these basic steps regularly will help you sharpen your capability to remember all that you prefer. Undoubtedly, practice makes flawless.

Methods for Kids

"Great things begin with little starter days." That is why, if you want to proficient at something, begin early. That is why if you have kids and you really want them to attain something in life in the future, begin now while they are still young. Specifically, with their memory, kids really need to begin early when it concerns memory improvement so that they would perform better in school and in the future. I know that we have all skilled memory issues at that time and the majority of the time, it is not since we're dumb and dumb but more as we were not using our brains in a best way.

In table for the brain to work effectively, we should also know how to use it in a way that it would be boosted and made the most of. This is the secret behind memory methods. The majority of specifically with kids, if you teach them while they are young about the right approaches of using their brain, and teach them about the methods that would improve their capability to keep in mind and remember things, they would be a lot more effective in remembering and remembering info in their head.

Every day, kids soak up countless information and info about every little thing. In school, the success rate of a kid in a school venture greatly depends upon how well their capability is to shop, procedure and remember the info that they get. Intelligence itself is based upon how well you pick up info and how effective you are in obtaining that info when needed.

There are some strategies that you could teach your kids so that they could enhance their memory while still young. Among these methods is what we call the "visualization and association." This technique is used by a lot of people who want to enhance their capability to remember. This is not a brand-new strategy or brain upgrade; it's just a technique of how to remember things in a lot more effective way. For instance, rather than remembering the word "light saber" you imagine the image of the light saber itself.

It is a lot easier for your brain to shop and recall "images" or "visual info" than spoken and written word. Images are concrete when they enter your head. That clarifies why you remember images more than you remember words. You may remember the image of the home and the street more than the name of the street itself.

So if you really want your kids to have a brilliant future, provide the right tools and you could begin by boosting the way they use their brain and you can be sure that they would be better residents in the future.

College and Profession Success

When you loaded for college, you most likely didn't forget your preferred outfits, music and devices. But to be successful in college and beyond you need to remember that memory abilities play an vital role in your success.

The human brain can make a record of and save unlimited info, but if you want to obtain this info you need to build your recall abilities. No matter how clever you are, learning is really reliant upon memory. Here are 5 memory strategies that will help you be successful throughout and after college.

1. Make a dedication to keep in mind.
You need to be encouraged to be successful and have an intent to keep in mind otherwise learning can't occur. How is it that a mixed drink waitress can keep in mind the beverages ordered by each consumer at tons of tables when brand-new people keep being seated all night? The waitress plans to keep in mind till the consumers leave. The waitress rapidly forgets the old orders so she can pay more attention to the brand-new ones.

In order to keep in mind the info you learn in college (at least till you have passed tests on it), you need to present the psychological energy to concentrate on the info you want to learn and ensure you comprehend it in the very first spot.

2. Organize the info you want to learn.
Remember when coming across info you want to keep in mind. Cluster the info in significant groups or classify products by value. Do not depend on recalling info you have heard if you do not write it down.
Keep in mind taking designs differ commonly, so use whichever style you choose. But you need to remember as an important step to bearing in mind what you learn.

3. Recite aloud to help move essential info from your short-term to your long-lasting memory.
If a stunning girl yelled out her contact number as her automobile scampered, an interested guy would most likely say the number over and over consistently till he could doodle it on paper. This exact same ability can be employed to learn the realities and figures you want to keep in mind.

Recitation works since it actively includes not only your mind, but also your body as it reinforces the neural trace in your brain.

4. Develop mnemonic gadgets where you appoint words, expressions, sentences or rhymes to difficult-to- keep in mind concepts or truths.
This is how we learned the notes on the lines in the treble clef: Every Great Kid Does Great or HOUSES for the 5 great lakes: Huron Ontario, Michigan, Erie, Superior. Mnemonics serve us for the rest of our lives when we want to remember info like how many days there are in a month:
Thirty days hath September, April, June and November.
All the rest have thirty-one, Other than February alone.

5. Picture what you want to keep in mind by creating a story or circumstance around it.
This technique of using images is called loci from the Greek and Roman orators who wanted to remember long speeches. To keep in mind the worlds in order develop a story about every one and psychologically tie it to the design of your home, for instance. Then take a psychological walk through your home getting each world as you go along.

These 5 strategies cannot work alone. They should be paired with great note taking, time management and selectivity. Nobody can keep in mind every little thing, so you need to be selective and learn to catch the bottom lines of the info you want to keep in mind. Then you should prepare your time sensibly so that you can disperse your memory strategies with time.

By following these memory methods, you manage what you keep in mind guaranteeing yourself a location amongst effective university student and profession specialists.

Learning a Foreign Language

Learning a brand-new language can be an uphill struggle. But if you use these basic memory exercises/techniques you could be begin learning a brand-new language in no time.

Memory method A: The One Hundred Words
The idea is that you only really need 100 strong words to cover over 50% of all words used in a discussion. By learning those 100 strong words you are one step ahead in speaking a brand-new language or at least perform a fundamental discussion.

But what are those 100 strong words? It depends upon the language and yourself. It depends on you to choose the strong words since each individual a figured out and/or is impacted by words in a special way. You can produce a list of words and keep including words to the list. Start with the 10 very first numbers from one to 10. Then include words you use really usually. You should find the hundred leading words of your daily vocabulary.

After you have completed your word list in your native language jot down the words from the foreign language beside the words from your native language. Workout on learning/memorizing the brand-new words and you will see considerable enhancement in the way you speak to other ones using the foreign language.

Memory strategy B: The Mnemonics
The idea behind this strategy is to use images to connect words between your native language and the foreign language. What you do is to associate all words with images in your mind. Then you begin connecting words by linking images and develop brand-new.

Here's an example of how to develop pictures of words in your mind:
You want to learn the Greek word for the English word "Eagle". First you imagine an eagle opening its substantial wings and flying over the mountains. After creating that image in your mind it's time to take a look at the Greek word which in this case is "Aetos". When you read/say the Greek word, try to envision the exact same image in your brain, the among the eagle flying through the clouds. That way your brain will quickly produce a connection between the brand-new word and the image of the eagle. This method will

help you learn and keep in mind brand-new words successfully and quickly.

Memory Method C: The Environment Mnemonic
This technique is rather advanced and is based upon the simple fact that the fundamental vocabulary of every language is in some way connected/linked to daily things in your environment (You should specify your environment, whether it is a space, a home, a town, a city etc). You should begin with a place/location you recognize with. The idea is to begin linking words with objects/locations in your environment.

For instance, you could associate in your mind the word "Library" with a picture of the public library and the word "Reserve" with pictures of the books inside the library. You could associate the word "Park" with a park in your town and the word "Tree" with the trees in the park.

This technique is so fun and simple when attempting to develop expressions by utilizing a mix of the above memory methods. You could quickly develop a picture of an expression like this one ". I went to the public library to get a book and after that I went to the park to check out the book.

Having a Long-lasting Memory

The mind is really efficient in growing and creating beyond what we give it credit for. Elderly people can significantly lower their brains do not have of focus by taking some time for little brain stimulation sessions every day.

It is advised to begin your brain workout 5 minutes a day, Monday through Friday and slowly developing to fifteen minutes a day session. The goal of the brain sessions is to only concentrate on the minds development by extending it beyond its regular though capability.

Brain methods can include anything that promotes the mind beyond its regular thinking capability. A great spot to begin is number memorization. The great feature of number memorization methods is that it is basic and really simple to chart development. It is also ideal for brain stimulation since numbers aren't relatively plain and not sidetracking. When doing brain stimulation, you do not want to be in the creative, visual mode.

List about 3 to 5 numbers on a paper. Now turn the paper over and see if you can remember what numbers you just wrote. Usage thicker paper so you cannot see the opposite side. Now include an extra digit till your brain actually needs to extend to bear in mind them all. This is where the advantage results.

Do this for about fifteen minutes a day, 5 days a week and you will start to see extra focus capability and memory strength. These 2 possessions work together.

You might include other workouts as long as they do not sidetrack you. Keep the objective of your workouts mind resistance and not increased intelligence. Work your mind out just like you would a muscle.

Now that you comprehend the fundamental concept behind memory strategy with a workout technique readily available, you can begin to arrange 5 minutes of your day aside for this alone. You will be surprised how much this little workout can help your capability to focus and keep in mind.

Loci's Approach

The word loci originates from the Latin word locus, which means spots. The method is also described as the memory palace. The strategy is an older mnemonic gadget. Allot of memory champ's use the loci technique. You do not need to be a genius to use the loci technique. It's in some cases described as the psychological walk. Various people use the system to keep in mind different things. Some want to remember wish list and other ones birthdays or faces. How does it work?

If you want to use the loci technique, you'll initially really need to choose a 'memory palace.' The memory caste can be the home you reside in, the city you reside in, and even just a product. There's only one thing you really need to make certain, you really need to know the memory palace by heart. See the spaces and products plainly in your mind. You're going to use this memory palace to keep the memories you really want in such a way that makes them simple to remember.

Start by acquainting yourself with the memory palace. You should see it plainly and strongly. It's essential that you have the ability to picture it. Make a path that you're going to take through the memory palace. If it's your home that is your memory palace, make a path that you'll take through your home. That you'll take through the spaces in your home. Envision every little thing as finest you can.

The loci technique works by associating the info you want to remember with a space in your memory palace. Want to keep a wish list? Imagine the very first product on the list in the very first room. Picture a bag of beans. Picture it plainly. It is inadequate to just see it. Action and feelings will make the info much easier to save. See the bag of beans increase in flames. Make it big. Include something to the image that makes it much easier to bear in mind. An example of a feeling I usually use is disappointment. I try to open the bag but can't, so I feel really annoyed and upset.

Spot the products you wish to keep in mind in the different spaces. The 2nd product on your wish list would enter the 2nd area. The essential element of getting this memory system to operate correctly is having a clear visual psychological image of the products, and to know your memory palace by heart. You will really need to come up with your own action and feelings to save the info. To be able to keep a whole deck of cards, you'll really need 52 places. Practice makes master.

Accelerated learning

Sport ability memory is developed when professional athletes learn and keep in mind motor abilities. Motor memory strategies can speed up the ability acquisition procedure so professional athletes can advance to higher levels of sport efficiency quicker.

Motor learning concepts are drawn from psychology and applied to sports training. Coaches can use the following sport memory strategies to accelerate ability learning and retention for professional athletes of any age:

1. Help professional athletes learn abilities properly the first time. Preliminary learning is most impressionable. An ability learned improperly is typically challenging to re-pattern. Coaches should keep track of and direct professional athletes to learn appropriate strategy when professional athletes are still in the early phases of learning.

2. Teach ability rhythms first, and after that improve the motions. Professional athletes can learn and remember balanced motions quicker than separated motions, just as rhymes are quicker recalled in spoken learning.

3. Portion motions. Motions can be learned and processed if they are "chunked", or organized, into bigger motions. This grouping method increases a professional athlete's capability to learn and perform sport abilities. Break abilities down only as much as essential. Over analysis triggers paralysis.

4. Make brand-new abilities significant. Clarify and show brand-new abilities so that the professional athlete comprehends what the ability needs and why it is carried out that way. Also explain how an ability, movement, or method will help the professional athlete enhance sport efficiency.

5. Associate brand-new abilities and principles with well learned abilities. Professional athletes learn brand-new abilities quicker if essential motions make a lot of sense to them. A coach can take advantage of a professional athlete's former experience and maturity level by recommending psychological images that associate brand-new ability ideas and functions with familiar ones.

6. Explain particular hints that need the professional athlete's attention. Intent to bear in mind notifies a professional athlete to essential elements of an ability or game circumstance. A professional athlete's capability to focus and keep in mind crucial hints differentiates novices from knowledgeable entertainers.

7. Overlearn abilities to right mistakes. Overlearning ways practicing abilities beyond what is required to perform them appropriately. It works for remedying formerly learned mistakes and for strengthening correctly collaborated motions.

Sport memory methods just like these can enhance training, saving important effort and time. These are just a few of the many tools used for how to successfully communicate what abilities and methods professional athletes really need to know.

Improve Your Focus Skills

One doesn't result in the other when it concerns memories and concentration. Your memory is your capability to keep in mind people, experiences and info. When you focus you direct your psychological powers and efforts to a particular, subject, activity or issue. You can learn abilities that can be learned to boost both concentration and memory. Practicing these abilities can boost success as a student.

Once something is saved in our brain, we always remember it. Nevertheless, we might have problem remembering the info; great concentration will also boost memory. If we only practice abilities that enhance our memory but never ever take a look at aspects that boost concentration, our efforts will only be partially effective.

A strong memory depends upon the health and vigor of your brain. There are a lot of things you can do to enhance your memory and psychological efficiency.

Workout
Your capability to keep in mind will increase if you can support your brain with healthy routines, as workout increases oxygen to your brain.

Sleep
When you're sleep denied, your brain cannot run at its full capability. Imagination, analytical capabilities, and important thinking abilities become jeopardized. Research shows that sleep is required for memory combination, with the crucial memory-enhancing activity taking place throughout the inmost phases of sleep.

Brain food
Just as the body needs fuel, so does the brain. A diet plan of "brain food" is based upon fruits, veggies, entire grain, and "healthy" fats. In addition to all the advantages of a healthy well balanced diet plan it can also enhance memory.

Brain Health club
Complete psychological workouts and activities that break your routine and obstacle you to use and develop parts of your brain that get neglected. Your memory is a lot like your muscles, it needs you to "use it or lose it." The

more you exercise your brain, the higher it's capability to keep info.

Friends and Fun
Make time for good friends and fun. Research studies show that a life that has lots of good friends and fun features cognitive advantages since human entities are highly social animals. We're not meant to prosper in seclusion. Our relationships promote our brains, implying communicating with other ones might be the best type of brain workout we get.

Research has revealed that a strong support group and significant relationships are important not only to psychological health, but brain health. There are a lot of methods to make the most of the brain and memory-boosting advantages of interacting socially. You can join a club, go to good friends, volunteer, hang out with good friends or connect over the phone. And if a human isn't readily available, a highly-social animal will do from time to time.

Tension Check
Persistent tension can damage brain cells and harms the hippocampus The hippocampus is the area of the brain where brand-new memories are formed and where we choose the retrieval of old ones. Research studies have revealed that meditation can help enhance imagination, learning, focus and concentration.

E-Learning

While it is really true that people continue to learn and get brand-new knowledge for as long as their psychological professors are working well, there can be circumstances when soaking up brand-new info and knowledge is not as easy a job as it would generally be. This is primarily just because of some elements that might prevent the absorption procedure, just like tiredness, tension, state of mind swings, age, and even injury.

The tension of daily living today has been reported as even greater than that of some years back, crediting to the tons of diseases and conditions typically credited to contemporary threats, just like progressive or unusual amnesia, or perhaps the failure to keep info and memories for long. This condition is especially obvious in members of a business's labor force, particularly those associated with high tension circumstances, those who might have suffered some form of injury, and those who might be thought about of innovative age. To continue being a reliable and effective member of the labor force, staff members should have the ability to update their ability whenever there is an important need to do so, or whenever their jobs and projects need them to do so.

The job of making sure that staff members have the ability to keep knowledge and abilities they learn is left to the training department, which in turn, utilizes e learning, to help in the job of making certain members of the labor force are undoubtedly able to continually operate well. eLearning uses the most ingenious mentor and learning strategies combined with tried and tested techniques to make sure that the shipment of the brand-new knowledge and abilities to the student is simple and reliable, and also simple to keep and remember whenever they really need it. E learning modules are structured to provide the most knowledge in the least amount of time, with learning modules structured to be simpler to keep and remember, which is just one of the more crucial aspects of the process.

eLearning uses some methods to enable students better memory retention in the learning modules, consisting of:

Info pieces - modules and subjects are bunched according to classifications, significance, and other groups, allowing for better retention through association. By organizing in certain lessons, the "memory chain" is more enhanced enabling an easier remembering procedure. An easier remembering procedure enables a nearly automated memory recall, by just focusing on a specific group, the needed info is remembered.

Rationally structured modules - frequently, the problem in remembering memory occurs from learning modules and lessons being haphazardly ready and structured, barely making any sensible sense of connection at all, making recall rather harder, since a ton of the remembering procedure uses attribution and sensible sequencing of ideas. E learning modules are structured in an extremely organized way, with appropriate series and links to consecutive lessons, to enable better recall and much easier retention.

Usage of sensory hints - an element of idea is that it usually includes parts that associate an idea with sensory stimuli, just like an image, a smell, a feeling, or a noise. By linking the idea or idea or lesson with a sensory hint, the mind has the ability to better shop the info or lesson, since the sensory hint ends up being a "tag" of sorts, enabling the student to efficiently link the sensory tag with the memory, and after that use the "tag" to remember the memory later.

Remember Things Much Faster

The human brain can more than many people even imagine. We keep in mind crucial things, and forget lesser things, but the simple fact is that even the lesser things are still kept in our minds someplace, stacked among the huge volumes of information in our individual disk drives. With a little practice and some used strategies, it is possible to learn how to remember quickly and keep things "indexed" so that you can obtain them anytime you really want. Let's analyze 3 of the well-known memory methods that can teach you how to remember quickly and effectively.

Associative Memory Methods: These kinds of memory methods include using really conventional attributes of our memory to help us remember quickly. With an associative method, a widely known product is connected with a just recently come across product as a way of creating a simple path to the lesser-known product for later retrieval. Popular associative memory strategies are mnemonics, connected lists, peg words, and a strategy called "psychological journey".

Visual Memory Strategies: With a visual strategy, psychological images is applied to practice a memory and produce a visual memory from this wedding rehearsal, even for a product that has no visual attributes. An example would be recalling an individual's name by drawing a visual image of what that name would appear like if it were an item, which will stick better in the mind since things are more quickly remembered that abstract ideas just like names.

Repeating: The majority of us are rather acquainted with this memory method, as a technique for studying for an examination in school. Repeating a product over and over boosts the probability that it will be remembered, so this is a relatively apparent method that the majority of people practice at some time in their lives. Nevertheless, repeating requires time and is not almost the most effective way to remember quickly and successfully.

All of these methods are different, but they run on a comparable concept, which requires creating a memory and giving it a brand-new way of entering your mind, as compared to what you experienced the first time you experienced the info. The way to enhance your memory is to utilize among these methods to make a much deeper impression in your memory, which will make you remember it more quickly.

Steps to a Much Better Memory
There are 5 primary strategies that can be used to enhance learning and retention. These strategies can be used as a student to enable you to enhance retention of product, complete your research quicker, and remember it rapidly throughout tests. These strategies are called:

1. Technique of Loci.

2. Pegwords

3. Memorhymes

4. PQ4R - Sneak Peek, Question, Read, Reflect, Recite, Evaluation

5. The 5th step is the most crucial. Leave your butt and begin using the strategies.

The very first 3 techniques are systems to enhance memory and recall. The 4th is an introduction approach that is used to totally engage the mind to bear in mind the product studied.

The very first of these approaches is called the "Approach of Loci," or in plain English, the Place Technique. It is also referred to as "The Memory Palace." As the title shows, this approach includes matching products to be remembered with a well-known area. Basically, you would envision yourself walking through a really familiar location (the roadway to the shop, the numerous spaces of your home, etc) and position the products to be recalled in each area.

This kind of memory strategy is revealed grippingly in the Hannibal Lecter books by Thomas Harris. In it, the lead character, the wicked Dr. Lecter, has the ability to flawlessly remember incredible quantities of info using the Memory Palace strategy. Nevertheless, you do not need to be a bloodthirsty genius to use this technique.

This is normally done as a sensible development or journey, For instance, on your typical walk to the shop, you would pass your front door, the mail box, the newsstand, Baskin Robbins, and so on. In your creativity, put a product from your list to remember in each place. For instance, if attempting to remember essential dates for a history examination, you could put them in the correct time series by having the Gothic War of the Roman Empire on your doorstep, which is naturally right before the starting of the Byzantine Empire at your mail box, which is naturally right before the High Middle Ages at the Baskin Robbins.

The strength of the technique is that our brains are better organized to save areas than random realities. Taking a trip through these places, as you would when giving somebody directions, is something we do naturally.

The technique to this technique, and undoubtedly all of the techniques covered, is to learn to use it rapidly and regularly.

Here are the steps needed to use the method:

1. Choose an extremely well recognized location, either your home, school, or other spot you are totally acquainted with. It is also crucial that the structure for your memory palace include spots you can move through. Keep in mind, we are attempting to use the part of your brain that is included with places and movement. The journey is important.

2. Next, list the functions of the path you have just chosen. As in the example above, the front door, the mail box, the shop; all appear in a particular series as you travel. It is necessary that the functions be unforgettable. You should have at least 10 functions for the very first tryout.

3. How can you make certain you have the functions remembered in the right order? Note them on 3 by 5 cards, randomize the cards by shuffling, and after that lay them out in the right order as quick as you can. When you can set out the very first 10 functions in order, include another 5 functions. Keep in mind, the more hooks you need to hang your memories on, more you can keep in mind.

4. With the area or path remembered to excellence, it's time to learn to use the

method. This method is called a "Memory Peg." Every one of the distinguishing characteristics pointed out above is a possible Memory Peg. To keep in mind the products in order, you should use your visual memory to develop a remarkable (.) scene at that place. I find this the hardest part of the workout, but making the scene unforgettable is to make it stunning or uncommon. I normally use humor. For instance, keep in mind the old animation of 2 pigs screwing with the caption "Makin' Bacon"? I use that image to represent bacon in my grocery list. So I walk through my door, see the pigs, and know I need to purchase bacon. There will be a Humpty Dumpty on the mail box to remind me of eggs, and so on till the list is complete.

5. And finally, it is very important that you practice the strategy. Repeat the journey through your Memory Palace sometimes to seal the list in your mind. Take the journey up and down to see if heading out of series triggers issues. If it does, you know you will really need to spend more time on this technique.

This is an effective approach and is one used by many students who are considered having exceptional memories. A lot of kids uncover this approach by themselves. The disadvantage is that it takes some time to learn to use and much practice to flawless. You cannot discover it on Friday and expect to use it to study over the weekend for finals that begin on Monday.

This is the very first in a series of short articles on memory strategies. Check my site or this short article directory site for the follow on short articles that go over the other techniques.

Photographic Memory

There are a lot of photographic memory strategies said to be able to help you develop a photographic memory. There have been a lot of research studies demonstrating that eidetic memory, also called photographic memory, is doubtful. It is an unusual capability found in less than 10% of the population, and whilst you might not be born with this capability it is possible to obtain it. Lots of photographic memory methods help your brain by enhancing your capability to bear in mind info. Your research study practices also play a part in this, as different people learn in a different way.

Having a photographic memory has a lot of benefits which should not be marked down. Nevertheless, it is not needed to have a photographic memory to enhance your studying capabilities. It can be replaced with other approaches just like mind mapping, or developing an effective info classification system. Alternatives also consist of only taking down the bottom lines that each chapter or book is attempting to communicate and making certain you comprehend the ideas. Many people are uninformed that whilst a photographic memory is an excellent ability, it is not without its downsides.

Among the essential issues with having a photographic memory is that you tend to struggle with info overload, having actually been exposed to a ton of info that might be unimportant or unimportant to you. Needing to handle such great quantities of info means that you are less effective in remembering the particular info that is needed, and you might also have problems in forgetting things which are unimportant to you. Having a pretty good memory is not practically recalling, but about having the ability to forget.

Having said all that, if you are still thinking about developing a photographic memory, you should turn to direction on how to develop this ability. There are a lot of books readily available, along with tapes and DVDs that supply such guideline and methods. The human mind functions in a comparable way to a computer system's database, and it is necessary to find the right linkages to call the right info. People aren't created to be databases for saving info. Your memory must be used to remember info that matters, instead of just for saving functions. Remember that a really good educational tool should teach you about learning, and not practically recalling.

Who says that only mind freaks can have photographic memory? You absolutely can hear the oohs and aahs when the Mind Freak himself had the ability to draw for you an in-depth illustration of the whole city just after a 5 minutes helicopter flight. It is a true miracle how these people have the ability to keep in mind so well. Now, imagine if you have the precise very same power and capability. Would not that be amazing? Simply look through your books the hour right before you sit for your examination and you will certainly score a true miracle 'A'. Take a look at these 3 efficient photographic memory strategies for you that you can use and gain from.

Right before beginning, photographic memory needs some sort of practice and method too. So if you can't do it after the very first shot, do not quit. Give yourself a long time to get used to it too.

First, the link system is normally used to help you with all sorts of memory work. This is highly beneficial for remembering texts in the form of lists or tasks. So, let's say if you have a long wish list to bear in mind, try to get all the words and try to make it into psychological circumstance out of it. Example, if you are given a list of things - pink, t-shirt, cat, slippers, ironing and flowers make an image out of the by thinking about FELINE wearing a T-SHIRT printed with FLOWERS and so on. When you reach the last product, try to connect it to the very first. This brief psychological movie will help you to keep in mind successfully and rapidly.

The 2nd technique is to use the peg system. The peg system is used normally to keep in mind images in a series. This number-shape system will help you to keep in mind the series of images properly in a jiffy. For instance, you are given images of a pet dog, cat, mouse, elephant, antelope and giraffe set up in this series. To use the peg system, just connect a number to each image Example 1 pet dog, 2 felines, 3 mice, 4 elephant et cetera. At the exact same time, use your psychological circumstance to make the peg system work. Keep in mind to connect the animals to one another, by utilizing the exact same method as discussed in the link system.

The last method would include making use of the ever-famous mind mapping. Back in the school days, the mind mapping method is an incredibly well-known and highly motivated strategy. Nevertheless, with time, people choose to chuck this strategy away just since they are finding it tougher to use. Well, this naturally depends upon the sort of location you are planning to use the mind mapping strategy for. To use the mind mapping strategy successfully, just take the essential main picture of the principle and branch off info that relates. It may get messier as you pass, but it is an outstanding tool for organizing a hectic schedule or keeping big amounts of info.

Developing photographic memory is not that difficult. If you aren't born with this gift, then get sly and experiment with these tricks and use them. Your good friends will be stunned by your significant enhancement in your memory work.

Have you ever questioned why stars can remembering long stories? Like if you see the script for an entire motion picture, it's included tons of pages. Specifically, if you are the primary star, you would be having a ton of discussions, and if I was the star, the very first question on my mind is "how on the planet am I going to keep in mind all of that?" well, that is the star's job. Nevertheless, they have a memory strategy to handle that. It's absolutely nothing fancy, absolutely nothing costly, just a minor change in the procedure of memorization that shows to be efficient, as you can see.

Among these strategies is association. Why call it "association"? Well, from the word itself, the procedure is associating the words with images, enjoyable ones. Something that is remarkable or something that you are truly used to and you would always remember. This is as your brains have the propensity to block undesirable images out. When doing this, you should certainly use images that are vibrant, lively and has sense. These makes it a lot easier to bear in mind compared to the ridiculous ones. Also, using all of your 5 senses works. Try exaggerating that image in your mind and make it funny, that way you would always remember it.
Here are also some of the strategies stars use to make their memorization abilities much more powerful:

1. Recorder - checking out the scene or the discussion and tape-recording it on a tape recorder. And after that replay it one thousand times and listen to it.

2. Envelope - acquaint yourself with the script or the scene and after that get an envelope, cover that part of the scene yon your script and imagine the person's face while saying those lines and take a look at the script again if you did it properly.

3. Writing - copy and write the lines into a paper but do it in series.

4. Tune - include some notes on your words, like a tune. Recite the script in a sing - tune way. (I do not know if this would work).

5. Crazy Man Method - mumble the words to yourself. Do it as though you are talking with yourself. And obviously, you should also address yourself, that's how it is. Caution: you will look absolutely insane.

Well, it thinks that's all of it. You could also try integrating all of these strategies and form one incredibly strategy that makes certain you would be remembering each line. But if you actually would like to know how stars remember their lines, you should go inquire. I'm quite sure there is some star out there who would absolutely tell you something about it. Or you could even try using the web, Google it and find the answer. But to make your life much easier, just settle with these things. These are the strategies that have the greatest possibility and guarantee that stars use them.

Subjects You Don't Like

Improving memory strategies are most needed for examinations. This is specifically the case, if you dislike a subject or a subject but you still need to modify for it. School kids or perhaps grownups battle to tackle this issue. Here are some enhancing memory strategies which can help you enhance your memory for subjects you do not like.

1. Self-Affirmation
This is a really crucial thing to do right before starting to study a topic. You really need to tell yourself that the topic is intriguing and that you'll enjoy it. You really need to actually believe in yourself that you'll have the ability to understand this topic by its throat and pass with flying colors.

This might sound ridiculous for those who have not done self-affirmation right before. But it works.

When you repeat declarations to yourself and try to truthfully actually believe in these declarations, you'll find that your sub-conscious mind will actually believe it. It will not take long right before you actually really believe what you're saying to yourself.

By continually repeating positive declarations to yourself and thinking in them, you'll find that you are more inspired and fired up when you begin to study the product. You'll have an entire brand-new perspectives on the subject and your memory will enhance ten-folds using this strategy.

2. Comprehending the Topic
When you read the topic, begin with the start and check out right through it

till the end. The point is not to remember the realities in this reading. The point is to comprehend what the entire image is of that specific chapter. You really need to comprehend the product and how it works.

Once your brain comprehends the reasoning of the subject and it understands in general the subjects covered, then you can begin modifying seriously by attempting to remember the realities. This memory enhancing strategy is really effective.

Since your brain comprehends how things work, recalling the specifics is so much simpler. Whereas if you do not comprehend the subject and just try to bear in mind the realities, the modification procedure will hurt and inefficient.

3. Usage Short Breaks
This memory enhancing strategy works hand in hand with the 2 methods defined above. When people try to remember truths, they usually keep in mind the start and the end most plainly. The bit in the middle is the part that is most quickly forgotten.

The reason is that when we begin modifying, we have an interest in the subject so the start of the product can be quickly remembered. The product which you have modified at the end is also more unforgettable, since you're happier since you're almost completed modifying and plus the product is newest as it's the last thing you have read.

Now if you take time-outs like a 10 minute rest between every thirty minutes of modification, you'll find that you can keep in mind a lot more realities. You're totally making use of the capability to bear in mind the start and end of the product to a much greater benefit.

These 3 strategies are a start to help you enhance your memory. You really need to learn more on enhancing your memory and with constant practice of the methods, you'll be saving a significant amount of time recalling essential things.

Chapter 5: Determination and Persistence

How to Build Your Own Persistence

What is persistence? Since it might be easy to comprehend the self a bit, it is
when the persistence is added that it ends up being 2 words in one that really
need to be cleared and completely understood.
To be determined is to have a mind that is not quickly discouraged. It means
to have a willpower about a specific problem or product regarding how one
has chosen to pass it.
Self-determination for that reason is a way to stay inspired and influenced
throughout a specific circumstance or scenario or experience without quitting
or getting out of the boat till the target or aim of the procedure is achieved or
attained. It is an individual willpower to always be a winner and never ever a
loser. It is a win-win mindset and mind set.
How do you build your self-determination? There are certain methods but let
us begin by going over just among them.

Focus

That is one effective active ingredient and tool that can be used to build one's
self-determination. It is not that simple to preserve concentrate on something.
Can you imagine how many things have crossed your mind just within the
time you began reading this great info about staying self-determined? That is
how difficult it can be to preserve focus and keep going without reviewing an
objective or target that has already been set.
You just pay attention to how quickly all of us derail from our objectives and
dreams and targets to the point of finding it so hard to achieve something or
anything whatsoever it is that can be described as deserving a while. All of us
fall into this loophole really quickly.
To conquer this difficult obstacle and stay focused in life about all that might
be our objectives and dreams and targets, we really need to have indication
posts and garden stays with gauge development in all that we lay our hands to
do.
The indication posts and development procedure bars also need to be easy
things that break down big and big jobs into littler bits so that it is a thing of
delight to celebrate every advancement point of accomplishment. This is
extremely essential in keeping focus and it eventually help to enhance our
self-determination.

Anybody can discuss how determined they are in the mind till they experience some interruption they did not prepare for and idea will only take several seconds or minute but wind up clearing them off their feet and floor covering their whole objective down the seamless gutter.

Preserving focus is not a simple job we should conclude but it is possible to accomplish it when the idea shared here is employed and appropriately carried out.

Once you use this idea of concentrating on little things along the way to great accomplishments, let us know how well it has helped you to attain your objective of building your self-determination both for the brief and long term.

Behind Every Success, there is Persistence

Yes, Decision! Decision!! Decision!!! A decision to be successful persistence to make an important difference persistence to carry on regardless of held up and errors.

Now, let us concentrate on ourselves, have YOU ever found yourself in a scenario where you really believed you would enhance your lot in life, only to find certain things that you didn't "register for"? Perhaps you began a firm or got a job that didn't begin well. Perhaps you were wed and things got difficult. My good friend, it's time I tell you this; Usually, in life, things get dreadful in some cases than you can imagine right before they get much better. Success I know is not a roller rollercoaster trip. There is a conspiracy going on that I want to expose to you here.

Know that right before you; a ton of effective people that we know today like Expense Gates, Oprah Windfrey, Tiger Woods, Jimoh Ibrahim e.t.c. have battled demoralizing obstacles that nearly tossed them off the ladder. But behind their great ideas, dreams, hopes, faith, imagination, and success was persistence. They were determined to get it through no matter what it will cost them. They were determined to get to the opposite side of life by creatively putting all they have got in them challenging their ugly circumstance. You know hardship can be uglier.

Like I said previously, there is a conspiracy going on between the 2 divides of hardship and wealth, effective marital relationship and divorces and so on. The god of success tests your willpower to be successful. They evaluate to see if you will be a really good ambassador of the success you are requesting.

It puts right before you the difficulties and difficulties to leap over. The majority of these difficulties are so frustrating that some people forfeit. Some people combat so tough that a minute to attaining success they pull out. But an identified person, the gods crowned.

For that reason, if you want to achieve success in this life, keep going, do not reverse simply because things aren't simple at the moment. Based upon what I have experienced, and studying the methods of great achievers, if success were simple, everybody would be doing it. No one will be blaming anyone for failures. The potential for achievement is in everybody including you, but to you have got be determined to work yourself through it. If you really want a result badly enough you will get it, but, you need to be determined to do what is required. Manage the difficulties of the moment in creative methods, but never ever reverse or forfeit on what you really want!

Getting Self-discipline

Self control is an individual's capability to manage feelings, desires and actions. It is the capability to separate the emotions from the self. When you let your emotions become you, your actions and choice making abilities become prevented. This might cause you responding based upon your emotions and not acting according to the circumstance. It takes a ton of practice and effort to get control over your emotions. But all that effort and practice will settle in the long run and lead the way for your success in leading a well-balanced life.

Requirements are different from desires. There are times when desires become so strong that they change into requirements. Self-control will keep those desires under control. Come up with your preferred food, and even better bring it home and do not eat it yet. As a primary step to self-control set your mind that you will not eat that food for 'x' number of days. I know, this sounds type of absurd, but believe me it works. Avoiding something that you truly crave for will develop resistance to impulses and desires in you. When you can withstand temptation, you have gotten control over your desires.

All our actions are specified by our feelings. Feelings are the hardest to manage, but if you can get that control over your emotions you have mastered self-control. Feelings could be anything varying from anger, joy, sadness, disappointment, and so on. Out of all these the largest step toward greater self-control is managing anger and disappointment. Anger subdues your mind and senses; you might do or say something that you will be sorry for later. Anger is self-destructive and you do not want to walk that course. When anyone or circumstance makes you angry/frustrated, try this: Count till 3 right before you respond or divert your attention to anything that will give the required time out right before responding. This time out will mellow down your anger, and as you keep practicing you will ultimately acquire complete control over your mood.

Meditation is just one of the best strategies to acquire self-control and stabilize your mind and body. Meditation helps unclutter your mind of undesirable ideas and feelings and also helps you focus and de-stress. Having a calm and clear mind allows you to manage your emotions and in turn your actions.

Anger Management Info

There is lots of appropriate anger management truths. Firstly, it is extremely essential to find out anger and the results of anger. Anger management will not work without understanding what it is a person is trying to change or manage. Anger is absolutely regular. It is a response to different situations. It is all right to be mad but when this anger ends up being extreme, frequently, there might be significant issues; issues within the family, bonds, work and it can lead to health problems. People who not able to manage their anger in a favorable way are very likely to move their anger to other circumstances like kid and spousal abuse, violent criminal offenses and other sorts of recklessness. This anger management information is just one thing an individual should think about when understanding they have an issue. There are all types of anger-provoking circumstances, more anger management details that may be of usage in resolving anger-related problems. Some people become mad or mad when they're disappointed, when something does not work out how they prepared or they couldn't prosper after giving their all, situations like these may lead to an individual to be irritated. This disappointment might result in anger that can then spin off into an entire list of negative consequences.

Inflammations provoke anger. Daily events like consistent pointers or routine disruptions can cause an individual to be exacerbated. This inflammation continues to grow and the outcome is an abrupt fit of rage. Depending on the person this rage can lead to an individual to turn to different methods of launching their anger, some of which might be painful to themselves and other ones.

When somebody is being verbally mistreated, maybe sexually mistreated, these circumstances provoke anger. Individuals handle these troubling experiences in a different way but for people who blow up just because of the abuse, the result could be truly serious, even violent. Anger management realities like this is vital, particularly in a circumstance where a private feels threatened. Being dealt with unjustly typically provokes emotions of anger. Frequently people are blamed for things, whether called for or not, it can trigger them to feel mad and act out as an effect of these emotions.

There is so much information crucial to comprehending anger management. The more truths an individual can collect, the better equipped they're when taking a look at situations including a mad person or if desperate to take advantage of the info themselves. Anger management specifics is available through tons of sources; books, motion pictures, in addition to the web. For a person who requires management realities, the web is an excellent source. With lots of sites devoted in management, it is extremely competent in providing the needed info needed concerning anger, effects of anger, people impacted by anger and anger management specifics.

Without the appropriate anger management realities, it may be challenging to start a kind of treatment that would be beneficial. It's trivial where the anger management specifics originate from. It does matter nevertheless; what a person finishes with the truths they're given. Checking out and studying the information is necessary but choosing what to do with this info will make the primary distinction in solving anger-related problems or not.

Anger Management and How People Express Anger

The volcano is the person who blows up or appears. This is the person who quenches their anger for a while, till it ends up being way too much and they can't take things any longer. For instance, they will:

* Physically last out at people. They might strike their partner; they might get in a bar battle while intoxicated.

* Verbally blast people. For instance, they might be verbally violent to their good friends and really loved ones.

* Storm off. Throughout a discussion, they might be activated and choose to

leave the room in a huff and a puff.

We have either seen it in other ones or saw it in ourselves. As discussed previously, these are the people who generally get sent out to anger management counselling and connected with having anger management issues. Nevertheless, the volcano reaction isn't the only expression of anger.

Passive Aggressive Reaction

An actually typical expression of anger (that a ton of people aren't knowledgeable about) is the passive aggressive reaction. In modern-day society (unlike in cave-men times) it isn't socially acceptable to reveal your anger using the volcanic technique. Individuals will call you unsteady, needing anger management counselling and is usually the 1 reason people lose their jobs and relationships.

So what do people do when anger builds within them in today's world? They respond in passive aggressive methods. For instance:

* Quiet Treatment. You will expect the other person (whom you seethe at or picking as a scapegoat for your anger) to be a mind reader and technique you to discuss your issue that you have with them. Frequently people, who use this technique will mentally close down and exist in body but not in spirit.

* Chatter. Rather than resolving your problem with the person whom you are frustrated with. You will chatter about them to work coworkers, friends and family.

* Usage of sarcasm, humor or subtle put-downs. In some cases people will camouflage their anger or irritation with somebody using this passive aggressive technique. Particularly, subtle put-downs that are camouflaged as a joke. Typically your mindful mind isn't even conscious that you are irritated with the person when you are doing it. And this is when the passive aggressive propensity is employed (usually without you even understanding that you are doing it).

There are certain passive aggressive propensities that people utilize, these are just 3 actually typical examples. How are you being passive aggressive in the different regions of your life as a way of expressing your anger?

I Do not Judge

The most crucial thing to do here is not to judge. Simply because you have volcanic or passive aggressive propensities doesn't make you an enemy. No one is flawless and all of us reveal our anger in 1 of these 2 methods from time to time. The essential thing is that we comprehend and understand regarding why we are acting in this way. Real behaviour change comes through awareness.

From my medical experience, normally the person or partner who has a volcanic way of expressing their anger will come along to anger management counselling sessions (or be pushed along). As the sessions go on, they typically make the realisation that they aren't 100% to blame for the circumstance. What they find is that other people in their environment have anger management issues too. The primary distinction being that they are better at hiding their anger. Typically "their" way of expressing anger is through passive aggressive propensities. This piece of awareness does not move the blame to the other person.

Firstly it is very important to be able to acknowledge anger in addition to the impacts connected with anger. Anger management is worthless without any knowledge of precisely what it actually is an individual is actually attempting to change and manage. Anger is totally natural. This is a reaction to a range of scenarios. It is also OKAY for you to blow up. Nevertheless, if that anger gets severe typically there may be bigger problems - concerns in your home, crucial relationships and the job. Likewise it can lead to health problems. People who are unable to deal with the anger in a positive way will most likely direct the anger in another direction like kid or marital abuse and vicious criminal offenses along with other types of irresponsibility. All of the anger management details is obviously something an individual should think of if they know they have a problem with anger.

There are actually a range of anger-creating scenarios and a lot more anger management information that could be advantageous in resolving anger-affiliated issues. Many individuals get upset or perhaps mad if they are irritated, if anything doesn't work in the way they meant or perhaps if they did not recognize success when they did their finest. Circumstances like these may trigger a private to get irritated. That irritation might lead to anger which could turn right into a whole set of negative results.

Agitation triggers anger. Every day circumstances like constant demands and typical interruptions might trigger a specific to get exacerbated. That irritation keeps developing till the result is an abrupt blasts of anger.

Depending on the person that disappointment might trigger a private to turn to alternative methods of releasing the anger, the majority of which may be undesirable for themselves in addition to other ones.

If an individual has been verbally maltreated, perhaps sexually misused, these scenarios triggered anger. People deal with these kinds of uncomfortable encounters in different methods. Nevertheless, for people who snap because of mistreatment, the outcome may be serious, actually vicious. Anger management information is certainly essential, especially in a circumstance in which a private starts to feel at risk.

Getting handled roughly frequently will trigger some feeling of anger. Generally, when folks are held accountable for errors, whether understandable, it might trigger them to become upset and also behave badly as a result of these experiences.

There is a ton of details important to comprehending anger management. The more details a person has the ability to gather, the much easier it will be to handle when they face circumstances that include an upset person or if maybe they want to benefit from the details themselves. Anger management information is offered through a ton of resources - publications and movies together with the Web. For someone that needs anger management details, the Web is actually an impressive resource. Having a ton of sites concentrated on anger management, it is exceptionally proficient at offering the crucial details needed concerning anger, results of anger, people affected by anger and also anger management information.

Without the appropriate anger management details, it may be tough to begin a treatment course which is handy. It will not make an important difference precisely where the anger management information stems from. It will make an important difference, on the other hand, precisely what an individual will do with the information they might be offered. Going through and also comprehending the details is important. Nevertheless, identifying how to continue using this details can make all the distinction in handling anger-affiliated issues or otherwise.

Bullying-Avoidance Methods

Avoidance techniques do not work as they do not remove the issue and they do not recover the problem. The issue remains and it continues to impact you. This certainly applies to all issues. The more you hide, the larger the issue gets. The more you run, the more the issue follows you and the larger it typically ends up being in your mind till you feel helpless to fix it.

Bullying continues till you make it stop or till the people bullying you choose to stop.

They might stop if, or when, another person - an onlooker or an adult [or group of either] tell them to stop. They might stop of their own accord. But they might not. They may feel they have no reason to stop.

They might well have ended up being comfortable in their role. It might have ended up being regular for them to bully and for you to play the 'victim.'

They may feel you have not provided any reason to stop. They may feel they are acquiring something from the circumstance, for any of the reasons noted formerly.

You need to organize the circumstance and make the bullying stop. You need to make it unrealistic for the bullies to continue harming you. In order to do this you really need to very first acknowledge that they are harming you.

This needs you to take a brand-new mindset toward the issue. I will tell you how to develop this in the future in the book.

Right before that I wish to take you through some of the 'Avoidance Methods' that people generally use in reaction to bullying.

Rejection

It's far much easier to pretend that the bullying isn't going on than it is to face it. People deny the issue to themselves and to other ones. They deny as bullying can be extremely frightening. To even admit that you are being bullied can be very challenging.

I also keep in mind several events from my own experiences where grownups gave me the chance to reveal the issues I was going through and I keep in mind plainly that I did not take those chances. My worry, my embarrassment, my humiliation, my sensation of powerlessness all held me back.

Instead I comprised some excuse as I felt embarrassed at feeling afraid and didn't really want anybody to know the strong pain I was in. When people did ask if I was okay, I would smile and say yes. In some cases people did defend me, but instead of use this as a springboard to change my thinking, I went on to deny the issue to myself and other ones. In doing so I cut myself off from the assistance I could have needed to sort the circumstance out.

Whatever you are going through. Wherever bullying is occurring, I really want you to know that you are exceptionally lucky. There is a massive amount of assistance and assistance readily available for anybody on the problem of bullying.

Neglecting It

Youths are typically advised by grownups to 'neglect' bullying. In my experience, I do not really believe that neglecting bullying works.

What I believe grownups are attempting to say when they advise this is 'do

not really believe the important things that bullies say, do not enable their words to become your ideas or do not innerise it.' But what it actually means is 'secure your self-confidence' by neglecting the vindictive, nasty, snide, threatening, violent things a bully may say.
You should safeguard your self-confidence from the words that bullies, 'neglecting it' works as a long term method. Disregarding something nasty that is said to you just once definitely can work. But bullying is not about one-off events. Bullying is relentless and repeated and even if you are pretending to overlook the bully, by leaving, by not taking a look at them or reacting to them, they know that you have heard and have not reacted.
The simple fact that you are neglecting the event is most likely to motivate them to say the exact same things to you again and again. They might even make it their objective to continue saying things till you ultimately fracture and provide the psychological reaction that they really want.

Visualisation
This technique is more of an individual one in regards to how I tried to handle being bullied. When I was at school, visualisation ended up being an escape. I would fantasize or imagine being in other places while at school and in lessons and I would imagine having a very different life when I returned home. I would lie on my bed and imagine bullying circumstances. I 'd actually close my eyes and imagine or visualize them in my head. If something had happened to me that day, I 'd replay it as a movie in my head. Then I 'd modify it and change it and replay it with a brand-new ending, I 'd see myself altering choices than the ones I had taken. So rather than being hit, I 'd see myself fighting. Instead of taking an insult, I 'd watch and hear myself speaking out and see it working.
I found these visualisation's really practical at the time. They were an escape. I believe in some way they enabled me a release, they enabled me to make it through what I was experiencing.

But there was a drawback.
I didn't understand the impacts the visualisation's were having. What I didn't understand at the time is that visualisation is really effective and your body responds to what you are illustrating in your mind just as if it were real.
When you imagine circumstances in your head and practice it to the point that you become able to imagine things really plainly, you feel the feelings that represent these circumstances really strongly too. You feel the physical

impacts of the circumstance you are imagining - if you're seeing a battle, for instance, you experience the exact same physical responses just as if the circumstance were real. Your body releases adrenaline and you feel the exact same feelings - you feel huge quantities of anger or worry. When you repeat the visualisation over and over, you wind up flooding your body with adrenaline which is not healthy at all.

Immersion
Immersion is a method of sidetracking your mindful mind from the strong pain you are in. People do this in a range of methods. You may check out a book and actually lose yourself in the book - its story, its characters, as a way of temporarily forgetting the bullying circumstance or putting it out of your mind. You may also do this with schoolwork, or sports, or preferred activities. Anything that enables you to focus on something besides the strong pain of the simple fact you are being bullied.
But behind the diversion is a significantly unpleasant truth: the circumstance is still there.
People in some cases bully other ones. They immerse themselves in the act of bullying other ones to try and forget the strong pain of their own bullying circumstance. People immerse themselves in beverage and drugs, anti-social behaviour, all to take their mindful mind away [temporarily] from their strong pain.

But that real pain is still there.
Avoidance techniques do not work. The best thing you can do is face the circumstance.
Some youths become 'school phobic.' They stop participating in school or certain lessons or activities where bullying may happen. You can find yourself keeping away from certain people and circumstances.
But what happens through avoidance is that your world diminishes.

You diminish the potential of your world.
You restrict yourself and your potential to be happy.
Every method that you use to stay away from the issue permits it to stay and the longer it goes on the more it results and changes you and lots of these changes can be extremely damaging to your life.

Self-Discipline for Attaining Success

We already know that self-discipline is vital, but do we actually really need it?

We know about success tools, and we acquaint ourselves with a lot of helpful resources that lead us to success, so why do we really need self-discipline? All of us have objectives for tons of regions of our lives. Some of us really want effective relationships, some like to get more cash, other ones really want just joy in their lives and other ones look for better health with less weight. These are really common objectives, and we often flop or be successful in attaining them. The general question is: Why we do not accomplish those objectives? Why we do not ended up being effective in these objectives?

The general answer is: Absence of self-discipline.

Success needs time. It doesn't happen simultaneously. What you do today will identify the lead to your future. If you change your present, you change your future. If you eat a ton of pizzas and scrumptious food today, you will put on weight, and this will display in your future weight. If you spend more cash than what you make today, you will have less cash in the future.

Present steps figure out future actual results.

Self-discipline happens in your present which will result in your future. You can learn a lot of ideas and tools for your objectives, but unless you do something about it for these objectives, you will never ever become effective in reaching them. Practically all objectives really need efforts and connection. Self-discipline will allow you to get required efforts and connection. If you really need to reduce weight, you really need self-discipline - to name a few abilities- to eat less. If you want to make more cash, you need to discipline yourself either for more cost savings or for more investing. Self-discipline requires time, and so is success.

It is about making some sacrifices. Yes, often it means doing some tough sacrifices. Why do we really need to sacrifice for anything? Why not just take pleasure in the moment of time and do what we 'Love' to do?

Obviously, nobody will require you to do anything you do not truly want to do. Nevertheless, we sacrifice since all of us have worths and crucial objectives in our lives, and these worths require us to decide: either enjoyment or that objective. The 2 cannot be attained in the exact same time, for the most part.

Our lives have plenty of temptations: we have Televisions, great food, chocolates, computer games ... and so on. These temptations makes it harder for us to withstand having more fun and hence we overlook the more vital objectives in our lives. Practically all of us want to have a slim figure, but with these temptations around us practically all of the time, we lose that objective of a slim figure. Nearly all of us want to make more cash, but it is challenging to withstand, for instance, marked down travel bundles. In these cases, we truly really need self-discipline. It will enable us to concentrate on our objectives and go after them till we reach success. With self-discipline, we can work out better control on our instantaneous desires.
It is the distinction between what you feel and what you believe.
It is the borderline between your heart and your brain.
You might want to eat that pizza which was revealed on a television commercial, but your self-discipline stops you since you have an objective of weight control, and in this procedure it enables you to prosper in that objective.

It is a fantastic resource for success. Actually, tons of professionals really believe that it is unrealistic to reach success without it. According to Lou Holtz "Without self-control, success is unrealistic, duration." Research shows that business owners should have it to prosper in company. According Jerry Osteryoung, who had dealt with 3000 leaders, he observed that what prevails amongst the effective ones amongst them, is not their education or intelligence or training, but it is their high self-discipline. For students, research studies show that high school efficiency is connected to high self-discipline instead of to high IQ level. I had met a 21 years of age student who completed high school with straight A's. He went to medical school, only for one year and left. He did not finish his research study. He also refused any training or guidance. His IQ level was extremely high at 154. Definitely with his high intelligence, he did not really need any training for how to study. However, he absolutely needed training for why to study. He just did not want to study, and he did not finish his research studies in spite of his intelligence. He did not have any self-discipline for research study.
It is a practice found in effective people.

And it is a psychological practice. Effective individuals were set psychologically for self-discipline. They use it naturally and immediately. That way, it is not a very hard effort for them to do and use it routinely.

We know that success has a pattern and typical laws. We also know that effective individuals ended up being effective just by following these laws. Numerous specialists studied effective people for several years and wrote a lot of wealthy & helpful books about them. One top specialist in this field, Brian Tracy, declares that one primary ability that you really need to accomplish success is the resource of self-discipline. You might know tons of laws of success, and you might have a map for your objectives, but this map will not work if you do not work out self-control for your objectives. It is a truth that 97% of people do not write their objectives, and this by itself is a major challenge to success, but just by writing the objectives is inadequate unless it is integrated with self-discipline. It is your useful map for success. It is your real practical steps that lead you to translating your objectives into success.

Effective individuals have high self-discipline, and they use it without experiencing challenge. They see it, not as a pretty hard sacrifice or dull jobs to do, but rather as a kind of flexibility. Flexibility from reliance on other ones, flexibility from procrastinations, and liberty from self-limitations.

We really need it for all regions of our lives. It is gotten in touch with time management abilities. With it, you can better organize your time. It can result in self-confidence, self-confidence and self fulfillment. You will really need it also for developing spiritual development, self-development and meditation.

It is one significant resource to reach what you can, your potential.

Some people were born with high self-discipline. Nevertheless, most people do not have it, and it is possible for them to discover it. This learning can be in 2 kinds: by mindful tools which means by day-to-day workouts for a long time, for a month or so. Or by unconscious tools like hypnosis, which is more reliable and longer enduring. In either approach, the person can obtain self-discipline and will have the ability to finish his required jobs as needed.

The Advantages of Discipline

Discipline is not satisfying at all. It is not acceptable for your individual program, and it always ruins every little thing for you. You need to get up early in the early morning to go to work although you have been awake the majority of the night watching a film. And discipline says leave the late-night motion picture, rather go sleep and have a great night's rest. It is bothersome for you since you actually wanted to watch that motion picture that was so intriguing. Get up, gown up and appear they say. That is describing your job. How are you going to manage to keep your job if you go to work when you just feel like? So, discipline says control yourself and be trustworthy at work so that you can make an income and support your family.

If you were not disciplined when you were young, then you are considered invalid kids. Which is quite apparent, any moms and dad would disciple their kids as they the moms and dad likes his kids. So, in what pick up a moms and dad would discipline a kid if that kid cannot have what it wants all the time? I believe a moms and dad would do that to teach the kid obligation, respect for other ones, and that the world doesn't focus on the kid. And a moms and dad would continue disciplining a kid so that those kids will cultivate great practices understanding that there are repercussions of their actions, great or bad. So, if you have great routines and a really good discipline, then you will have great consequences. And the reverse will happen if you have bad routines. So, if your mother and father really love you, then they will discipline you as it is for your own great. When you are young, you do not comprehend this principle. If you are being disciplined you regard it as penalty, and you are uncertain why you are being penalized. But take heart, it is not that you are being penalized for absolutely nothing; your father and mother are disciplining you for your own great, so that you can flourish when you are older.

The best way to learn much from discipline is do not battle against it. Do not rebel against your father and mother; they are disciplining you for your own great. Deal with the entire disciplining procedure and do precisely what is expected of you. And do your tasks voluntarily, and your life would be more enjoyable. Above all, watch your mindset at all times. Work voluntarily with discipline and it will be more manageable and enjoyable for you. Work at your discipline; build a practice of keeping to the guidelines and policies of your discipline. Then, your discipline will not become a discipline any longer, since you do what is expected of you by practice. Discipline is simple to cope with, supplied you do not battle against it. And if you rebel against your father and mother and their discipline, you are going to have a most dog's life. So, begin early in life and cultivate a disciplined life. Beware of your mindset toward your moms and dad's discipline, the do so for your own great.

Strength Training is All in the Mind

What is strength training?
Strength training is carrying out workouts with the intent of making your muscles more powerful. These workouts typically take the form of carrying out a motion against a resistance, for instance your bodyweight or dumbbells.

How strength training is different to bodybuilding
Bodybuilding and strength training are usually erroneously considered being the exact same thing as they use comparable techniques, but there are some crucial distinctions in the training approaches, the end results and most importantly, the main aim. In bodybuilding, there is one objective: looks. The aim is to increase the size, meaning and balance of muscles to build a remarkably muscular physique. Bodybuilders increase in strength as they train, but this is only an adverse effects of their training. In strength training, the primary aim is to increase the strength of the muscles. Strength training will also tend to increase the size of the muscles, but not to anywhere near the exact same level as bodybuilding.

Elements impacting strength
In essence, strength is a procedure of the capability of a muscle to apply a force against a resistance. Although the size of a muscle is usually associated to its strength, one doesn't always follow the other. It is possible to enormously increase your strength without getting much, if any, muscle mass and it is also possible to increase the size of your muscles without acquiring much strength. Increasing muscle mass will increase your strength since you will have more muscle fibers to use a force. Nevertheless, when you raise a weight, you never ever actually use all the readily available muscle fibers at the exact same time. By learning to increase the number you use, you can increase your strength without increasing your muscle mass. The number of fibers triggered in the muscle depends upon the signal that they get from the brain When training particularly to get strength, your nerve system will learn to trigger a higher percentage of the muscle fibers, which increases your strength.

Training the brain.

If you want to get more powerful, you really need to concentrate on the nerve system as it is this that has a higher impact on your strength than anything else. Unsurprisingly, the best way to train your nerve system is to raise heavy weights. Increasing your strength is mainly about training the connection between your mind and your muscles. By applying big forces to raise heavy weights, your nerve system will learn to adjust to them. You really need to be raising weights such that you can only manage between 2 to 5 repeats per set. Any more than this and the weight isn't heavy enough. Training frequency also has a huge impact. For optimal strength gains you really need to train frequently and typically.

Many bodybuilding regimens train each body part only once each week to enable the muscles to completely recuperate. Strength training taxes the muscles in a very different way so the healing duration needed is not so long; it is mostly the nerve system that is being trained. You should be aiming to train each body part around two times a week. Strength training exercises should be brief, but extreme. You should not be training to failure. Training to failure will increase the time needed to recuperate, which will not help you get strength. Picking the right workouts is also essential for building strength. The most efficient types of workout for strength are heavy substance lifts and bodyweight workouts. For instance, barbell squats and pull-ups.

Kinds of Strength Training
In many sporting circumstances is not the optimal strength important for enhancing efficiency.
It needs different training to develop muscle strength proper and practical in regard to the circumstances pointed out above. Farther, I for that reason take a look at some strength training approaches for the development of:
* The optimum muscle strength
* Muscle Volume
* Fixed muscle strength
* Doggy muscle strength

Training of optimal strength with a big external load.
If you want to do a muscle group so the bar as possible, you really need to both develop the sample of muscle and enhance neuromuscular function. Experiments have revealed that the best actual results if you use big loads. This means items that weigh between 80 and 100% of 1 RM (one repeating optimum). If you are raising so heavy, it is very important to be well trained

in advance. You should also master the body usage and have great lifting technique.

If you can stand more than 4 to 5 repeats per series, this is a great indication that you can increase the load rather. Want to get great actual results, you should work out at least 3 times a week, those who put great focus on this approach of training days are typically between 4 to 6 times a week. Keep in mind nevertheless that it is required to give the different muscle groups sufficient rest between exercises. Moreover, you really need to find workouts that "hit" the muscles of the different sport's needs. There is this thing called requirements or requirements analysis.

Training for optimum strength with medium-sized external load.

From scholastic quarters Mon advised not to begin working out optimal strength till 16 years of age. A beginner ought to not train with loads going up to the optimum. 50-60% of the optimum is heavy enough to offer a functional training influence in the preliminary adjustment stage.

If you are strong enough and have a great lifting technique, you can differ any of these physical fitness models in the bench press and squat.

Training of muscle volume - body structure.

The objective of a bodybuilder is to be as muscular as possible. In order to get developed a big and noticeable musculature on the body parts that are examined in body structure/ body structure, they need to eliminate excess fat and build muscle cross-section of extensive strength training with reasonably modest external weight loads. This can only be attained with a stringent diet plan (cutting) and a training program that develops the muscle percentages. The primary pattern is that this training be executed with lots of repeats (associates)/ series (set). "Pump Technique" is about this strength training form called.

Professionals actually believe that bodybuilders who train with fairly moderate weight loads, it will endure improperly in weight-lifting and powerlifting than professional athletes who train with external loads up to the optimum. This would then mean that the training approaches of a bodybuilder is less very likely to develop optimal power.

Body Home builders situated at a high level of efficiency, training approximately 2 sessions of the day the majority of the year. Every muscle group is generally trained 2 to 4 times each week. One exemption is abdominals (stomach) that they work out at least 4 to 5 times a week.

Training of fixed (isometric) muscle strength.
Practical experiment:
Lock a boom on the upper side, lie on your back and try squeeze all you can stand with their feet against the pole. You can sign up rapidly that there's something in the muscles that extend the hip and knee joints. If you push the optimum, you see that you only manage to claim a brief time.
Muscles that work in that way, carries out a fixed work. There's no movement in the joints while you are in, and muscle length doesn't change. Capillary in muscles compressed, and there is practically a loss of oxygen - energy profits is mostly anaerobic. The muscles become exhausted, and they will strengthen if the fixed muscle work lasts a while.
Concerning the requirements for stability and to preserve body position, this will differ from sport to sport. In some sports like shooting with rifle, handgun and bow, we look for the body positions and making use of muscles that supply the quietest of body and equipment. This is called the fixed stability. In other sports have muscles sustain a consistent fixed pressure (where the external force variations are quite foreseeable). Such fixed stability is required eg. of the lower arm muscles/ fingers in connection with windsurfing (keep the boom), and the thigh and seat muscles that hold body position steady in speed skating. The stability also means opposition to the fast and unmanageable variation in external impact, as in fumbling, judo and snowboarding there all the time are speaking about vibrant changes of body position relative to the surface area, lighting conditions, challengers, methods, and so on
. The fast variations in the external power pattern in these sports need great force to the speed of mobilization and power development with a view to supplying a vibrant stability. Similar to other strength training also use to fixed workout that you can advance as you train on. Training impacts the strength of the muscle length you train in. You develop optimal isometric strength by fixed workout with optimal effort. And you will be better to hold a long position, you need to train for long sessions.
The training of the optimum fixed strength, it is most convenient to deal with an opposition that is so great that you are unable to make some movement. Perform the workouts in different positions in the movement course. Using 3 different positions in the joint, so that you work out the muscles in 3 different preliminary lengths.
If you train endurance, fixed muscular strength for a specific sport, the

training must be made in relation to the requirements set sport when it pertains to tension, period and body position. In many cases it might work to integrate such training with the vibrant work. The following approaches might be proper for the training of endurance fixed muscle strength:
Model A -> Hold Time: 10-12 seconds (3-5 repeatings) x 5 series - breaks 1-2 minutes.
Model B -> Hold Time: optimum (one repeating) x 3 sets - 3-5 minute breaks.
Model C -> Hold Time: 10-12 seconds (10-15 associates) - 5-15 2nd stops briefly.
Training influence of optimum fixed strength heads out particularly to increase muscle sample. This training approach is to some degree used to supplement training in modern-day weight lifting. Training of consistent fixed muscle strength is readily available in the rehab or injury, for people who will train the supporting muscles in the abdominal area and back, or to stop muscle waste.

Training of muscle strength endurance.
With consistent muscle strength really believed to have the capability to muscle to save money power intake.
How much power we can develop over a fairly long period of time is vital in sports where you need to get rid of an external load or resistance lots of times. Such sports are canoeing, rowing, swimming, cross nation snowboarding, alpine snowboarding, skating, fumbling, cruising, far away and a lot of ballgame.

What to Expect in the Marine Corp Training

In the Marine Corp training, you are transformed from a civilian into a soldier. The employees are trained to endure chances and difficulties but people should know how to work within a group. The shared extreme experience is what produces comradeship and requirements of conduct so that Militaries will not let anything stand in their way.
The Militaries aren't only trained to be difficult physically but psychologically too. The Core Worths- Honor, Nerve and Dedication are what mold hires to be who they're supposed to be. What can you expect throughout the Marine Corp training?

You will have the longest and hardest 13 weeks of your life. In your hire getting stage, you will get your extremely first Marine hair cut. Your preliminary equipment will be provided and that includes your uniform, toiletries and letter writing products. Throughout this stage, you will have your full medical and oral screening and you would need to take the IST or Preliminary Strength test. This test would consist of a one and a half mile run, sit-ups and pull-ups. This is done to check if you are in shape to begin the training.

Next will be forming. What happens throughout forming? You will meet your drill trainers for the first time and throughout this 3-5 days stage, you will learn the fundamentals- how to march, how to wear the consistent correctly, how to protect your weapons and so on. You should have the ability to adapt to the training way of living right before the very first real training day.

What else is included in the Marine Corp training? You would need to go through the drill, physical training, scholastic training, core values, Marine Corps martial arts program, self-confidence course, battle water survival, fundamental warrior training, field training, marksmanship training, FFR, field meet, crucible, shift stage and last but not least, family day and graduation.

Leading Idea - Enduring Marine Corps Basic Training
clarify the leading suggestion for you for enduring Marine Corps fundamental training. Just one thing that you need to comprehend is why you need to go through standard training to start with. Standard training is established so that you will be broken down into a powerful challenger for the opponents in a wartime circumstance. In essence, you will be changed into an effective battling robot. You will no longer be a specific, you will enter into a really effective and strong system that will be flawlessly trained to combat and to make it through. Here is the best pointer that I can offer you with for preparing yourself for bootcamp.

Psychological Preparation Is Essential:
Comprehend that you have an inner capability to handle things that you never ever needed to handle in the past and that you most likely currently feel are unrealistic to handle. The brain is a remarkable thing, and actually you only use a part of our brain every day. Going through fundamental training, you

learn to handle circumstances that the regular person is not able to do with psychologically or physically. Simply put, my significant suggestion for you is that you should begin to prepare yourself psychologically right before getting to bootcamp to breeze through the training sessions.

This psychological preparation can be done in many methods. However, learning to practice meditation, to focus, and to focus on a level that you never ever needed to achieve formerly is a great strategy. Once you handle something psychologically through visualization, then the physical part will just be secondary.

How to Make Better Choices

Making great organization choices is an important ability that can be learned and used throughout your life. On the other hand, a bad company choice can impact and destroy you, your workers and even your company completely. In simple fact, bad organisation choices are among the leading reasons for overall business failure. Bad choices are usually made when we become mentally caught up in a circumstance or we just do not have the persistence required to make the clever choice. Great company choices need that you follow these significant steps; figure out the right technique, know and comprehend your alternatives, collect info, and comprehend the consequences. If you learn to always follow these steps as you overcome the choice making procedure, you will likely become an excellent choice maker throughout your life.

Step 1 - Identify the Right Technique: There are 4 typical approaches that are used in the choice making procedure; command, seek advice from, vote and agreement. Each features an increasing degree of individual participation and an increased dedication level. Nevertheless, more individual participation also reduces the choice making performance. If you will make the effort to learn and comprehend these 4 approaches of choice making and use them appropriately, you will be on the way to ending up being a great choice maker.

Command: The person in charge always makes the decision and the choice making procedure is usually made really quickly without much idea. This Process includes only the person in charge leaving all other ones to handle the choice whether they like it or not. This is a great way to decide if other ones aren't impacted by your choice and the possible effects are small.

Speak with: The choice maker collects info and viewpoints from other ones to help him/her make the decision. This includes more people and resources, but the decision is still made by the person in charge. This is a more considered and computed choice making procedure and is a great way to decide as long as other ones aren't seriously impacted. Can you remember other ones might not concur with your choice, so ensure you know when to use this procedure.

Vote: Members of the group use their viewpoint by voting for their choice to identify the decision based upon well-known choice. This is a great way to collect everybody's viewpoint to help you make a fast choice that pleases most of the group. Nevertheless, this will likely not please everybody, so if you are trying to find an overall group contract right before a decision is made; agreement is the right choice for you.

Agreement: Everybody is included and talks through the alternatives till everybody settles on an option or partnership of choices. A decision is not made till everybody in the group accepts a typical choice. This is a great way to accomplish organisation cohesiveness and group dedication, but it is normally really ineffective and can result in hold-ups in the choice making procedure.
Now that you have determined what choice making procedure is proper for your circumstance, relocate to step 2.

Step 2 - Understanding and Comprehending Your Alternatives: You can develop an easy list of choices with a little research and some brainstorming. This procedure will help you widen your thinking and open the door an universe of choices. After you have your list, develop a list of advantages and disadvantages beside each choice to help you limit your choices.

Step 3 - Gather Details: Investigating your alternatives and collecting info is just one of the most essential steps in making wise organisation choices. Better Company choices can typically be made when precise info and company data are readily available. If you can pull immediate sales, stock, monetary, worker and other crucial organisation reports and records connected to your business, you will have a great benefit in making great service choices. If you are not able to pull precise service reports that help you in the choice making procedure, we suggest an entirely free to try service management suite that can drastically help you become more effective at running your company and give you the abilities you really need to be able to pull important choice making reports.

Step 4 -Comprehend the Outcomes: With every choice there is a very good or bad consequence which is why it is so essential to comprehend the prospective result of your choices. You can use your benefits and drawbacks list from step 2 to help you get ready for possible results. Comprehending the possible results of your choices can help you be more ready to deal with any future circumstance that might develop.